THE
YOGA
WHEEL
BOOK

50 Poses

For Stretching, Flexibility, Strength and Posture

YOGA WHEEL CLUB

We hope you enjoy this book!
Please support our small, independent business by leaving us a review on Amazon.

The Yoga Wheel Book

The author and publisher shall have neither liability nor responsibility for any person or entity with respect to any loss or damage caused or alleged to be caused, directly or indirectly, by the information contained in this book or any related materials.

First edition January 2021
www.yogawheel.club
@yogawheel

Contents

Introduction 5
The Practice of Breathing 6

STRETCHES

Thoracic Stretch 9
Urdhva Dhanurasana

Crescent High Lunge 11
Ashta Chandrasana Pada

Spinal Twist 13
Vakrasana

Rolling High Lunge 15
Anjaneyasana

Revolved Head to Knee 17
Parvritta Janu Sirshasana

Cow Face 19
Gomukhasana

Revolved Forward Fold 21
Parivrtta Prasarita

One-Legged King Pigeon 23
Eka Pada Rajakapotasana

Fish Prep 25
Matsyasana Prep

Side-lying Fetal Hip Opener 27
Parsva Savasana

Half Standing Forward Fold 29
Ardha Uttanasana

Supported Bow 31
Dhanurasana

BEGINNER

Handstand Prep 33
Adho Mukha Vrksasana Prep

Warrior 35
Upavistha Virabhadrasana

Seated Warrior 37
Virabhadrasana

Double Leg Raise 39
Uttana Padasana

High Plank 41
Phalakasana

Half Moon 43
Ardha Chandrasana

Lotus Fish 45
Padma Matsyasana

One-legged Half Boat 47
Eka Pada Ardha Navasana

INTERMEDIATE

Fish 49
Urdhva Dhanurasana

Garland 51
Malasana

Dancer 53
Natarajasana Hasta

Locust 55
Salabhasana

Standing Backbend 57
Anuvittasana

Standing Forward Fold 59
Padangusthasana

One-legged Bridge 61
Eka Pada Setubandha Sarvangasana

One-legged Side Plank 63
Eka Pada Vasisthasana

Toe Stand 65
Padangusthasana

Side Bend with Butterfly Legs 67
Urdhva Hastasana

Bird Dog 69
Dandayamana

Upward Bow 71
Urdhva Dhanurasana

Seated High Lunge Backbend 73
Upavistha Ashta Chandrasana Backbend

Pike Handstand 75
Adho Mukha Vrksasana

ADVANCED

Dancer Balance 77
Natarajasana

Handstand 79
Adho Mukha Vrksasana

Bow 81
Dhanurasana

Scorpion Handstand 83
Vrschikasana

One-legged Upward Bow 85
Eka Pada Urdhva Dhanurasana

Floating Camel 87
Ustrasana

Headstand with Wide Legs 89
Salamba Sirsasana Konasana

Splits 91
Hanumanasana

One-legged Peacock 93
Eka Pada Mayurasana

Pigeon 95
Kapotasana

PARTNER

Bridge and Crow 97
Setu Bandha Sarvangasana and Bakasana

Half Feathered Peacock 99
Ardha Pincha Mayurasana Padanguli

Double Feathered Peacock 101
Pincha Mayurasana

Scorpion Handstand Prep 103
Vrschikasana Prep Uttanasana

Bridge and Standing Balance 105
Setu Bandha Sarvangasana and Pranamasana

Seated Meditation 107
Sukhasana

Disclaimer

Always consult a medical professional before beginning any new exercise programme. The information provided in this book does not intend to prevent, diagnose or treat any medical condition or disease. If you experience pain, dizziness or discomfort while attempting any of the poses in this book, please stop and consult your doctor. Any yoga practice involves the risk of injury. Yoga Wheel Club is not liable for any injuries or damages connected with the use of this book.

Introduction

The Yoga Wheel is a powerful tool that can transform your yoga practice. It can help you reach more difficult poses by improving your flexibility, posture and strength.

If you already practice yoga, the wheel can push you to reach more advanced postures and develop your practice. It's not just for experienced yogis though. If you are starting yoga, then the Yoga Wheel can act as a supporting tool to help you balance in your first poses and develop your strength.

This book outlines how you can use the Yoga Wheel to practice 50 yoga poses, with illustrations and instructions.

If you are new to the wheel, start with some beginner poses, before moving on to the intermediate or advanced sections. You can also try some partner poses to share the joy of the yoga wheel with friends.

Grab the wheel and begin your journey!

The Practice of Breathing

Pranayama

Before considering any of the poses in this book, it is important to be conscious of your breath. Deep breathing can calm and focus the mind, preparing you to challenge the body.

As you work into each pose, make sure to incorporate breathing practice to create stability and support your movements.

Breathe Deeply

Your breath should guide you through all movement. Your goal in each pose is to be comfortable and to breath effortlessly. You should feel relaxed in your breath and not under any strain.

How to Breathe in Yoga

Use this as a general rule to syncronise your breath with your movement.

Inhale during...

Backbends

Opening the chest

Raising the head

Raising the arms

Exhale during...

Forward bending

Twists

Side bends

YOGA WHEEL BOOK

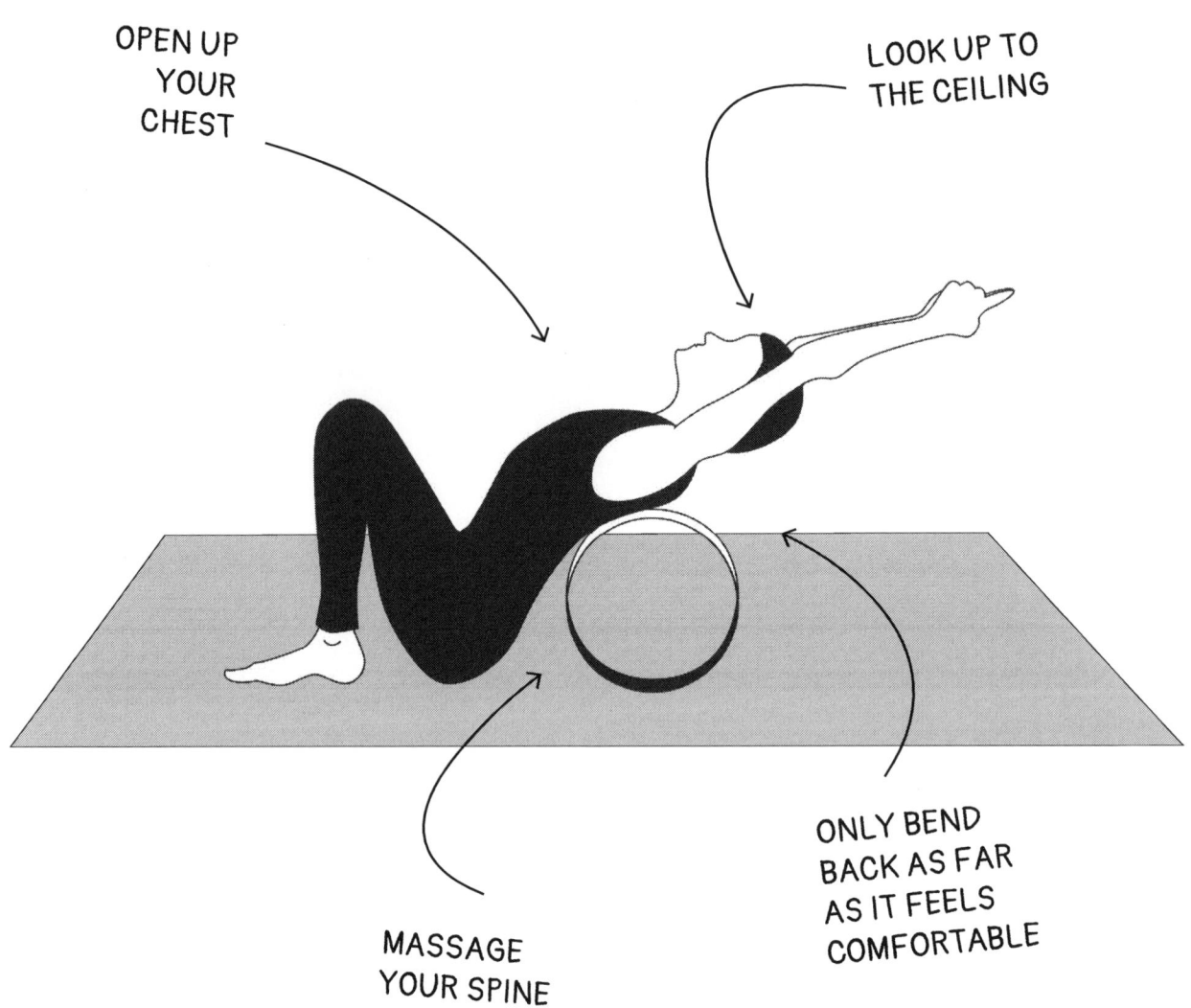

Thoracic Stretch

Urdhva Dhanurasana

The Thoracic Stretch is a lovely way to massage the spine and remove any tension in the back. It's the perfect antidote for poor posture caused by sitting at a desk all day.

1. Sit with your knees bent and place the wheel behind you in the centre of your spine.

2. Slowly bend backwards until your shoulders are resting on the wheel.

3. Stretch your arms above your head and look up to the ceiling.

TARGETS: SPINE, POSTURE

YOGA WHEEL BOOK

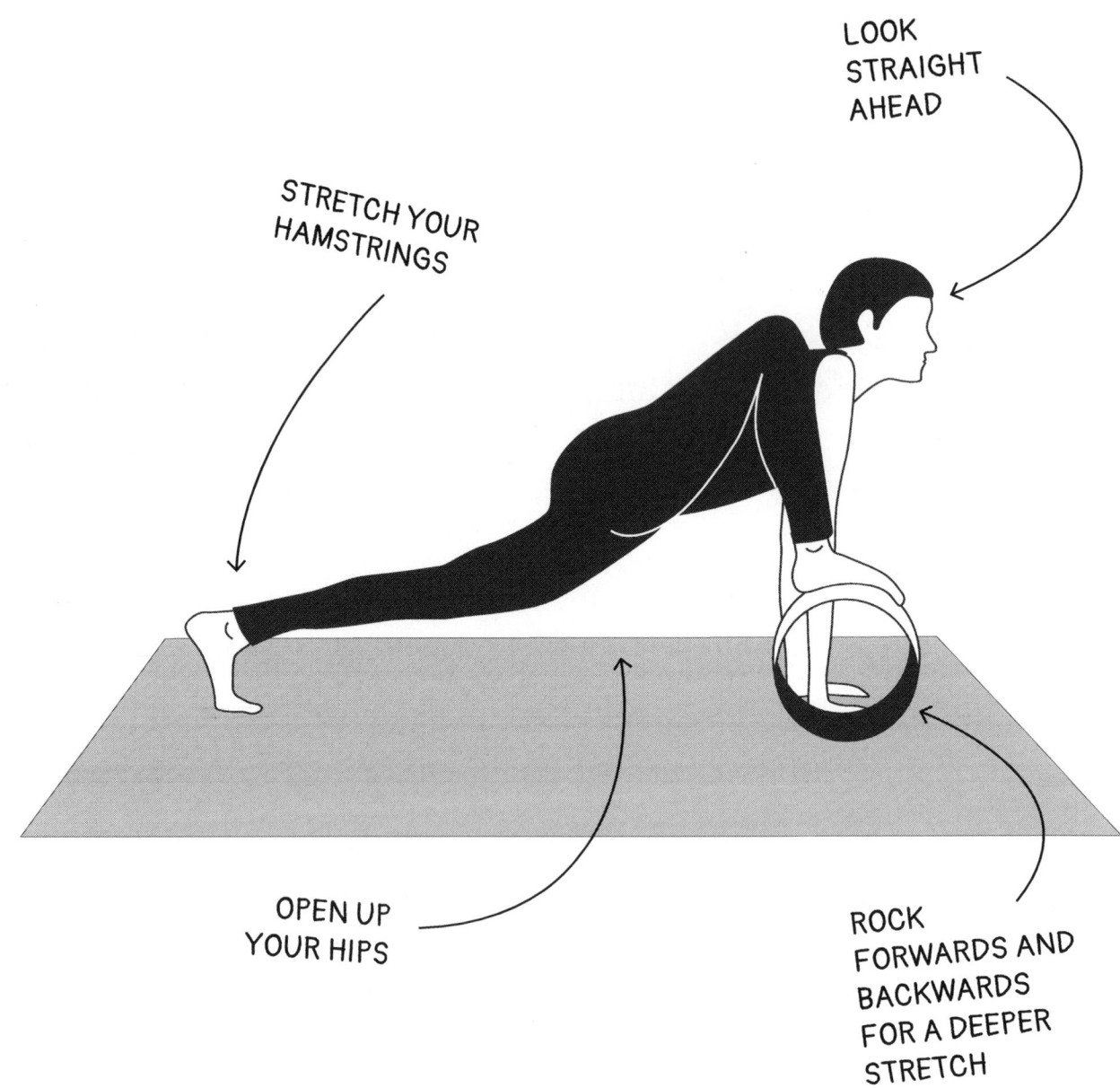

Crescent High Lunge

Ashta Chandrasana Pada

The Crescent High Lunge is an advanced stretch, that is perfect for opening up the hips and stretching the hamstrings. Using the wheel transforms this into a dynamic pose. You can achieve an even deeper stretch by gently rocking forwards and backwards on the front foot.

1. Begin in a high plank position, with the wheel positioned next to your right wrist.

2. Step your right leg forward into a high lunge, and then place the sole of your foot on the wheel.

3. Gently roll the wheel forwards and backwards to open up your hips, keep your upper body stable and look straight ahead.

TARGETS: HIPS, HAMSTRINGS, ARMS, SHOULDERS

YOGA WHEEL BOOK

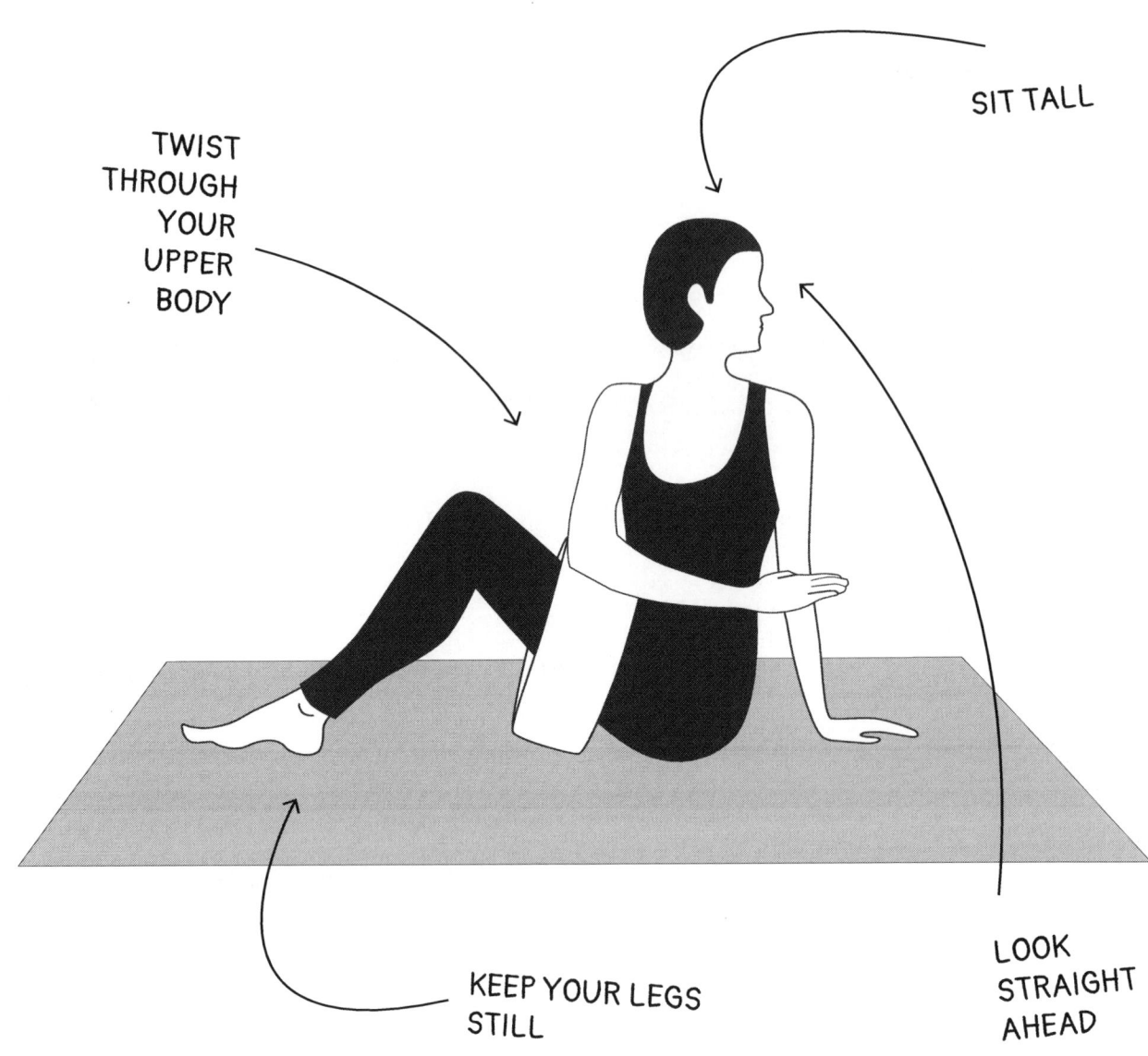

Spinal Twist

Vakrasana

The Spinal Twist focuses on rotation through the spine. Using the wheel helps to keep the legs still, allowing rotation through the upper body.

1. In a seated position, place the wheel over your legs and bring it up to your thighs.

2. Bend your knees so that the wheel rests on the floor, and then sit tall.

3. Place your right hand behind you and slowly twist your upper body towards your right side.

TARGETS: SPINE, POSTURE

YOGA WHEEL BOOK

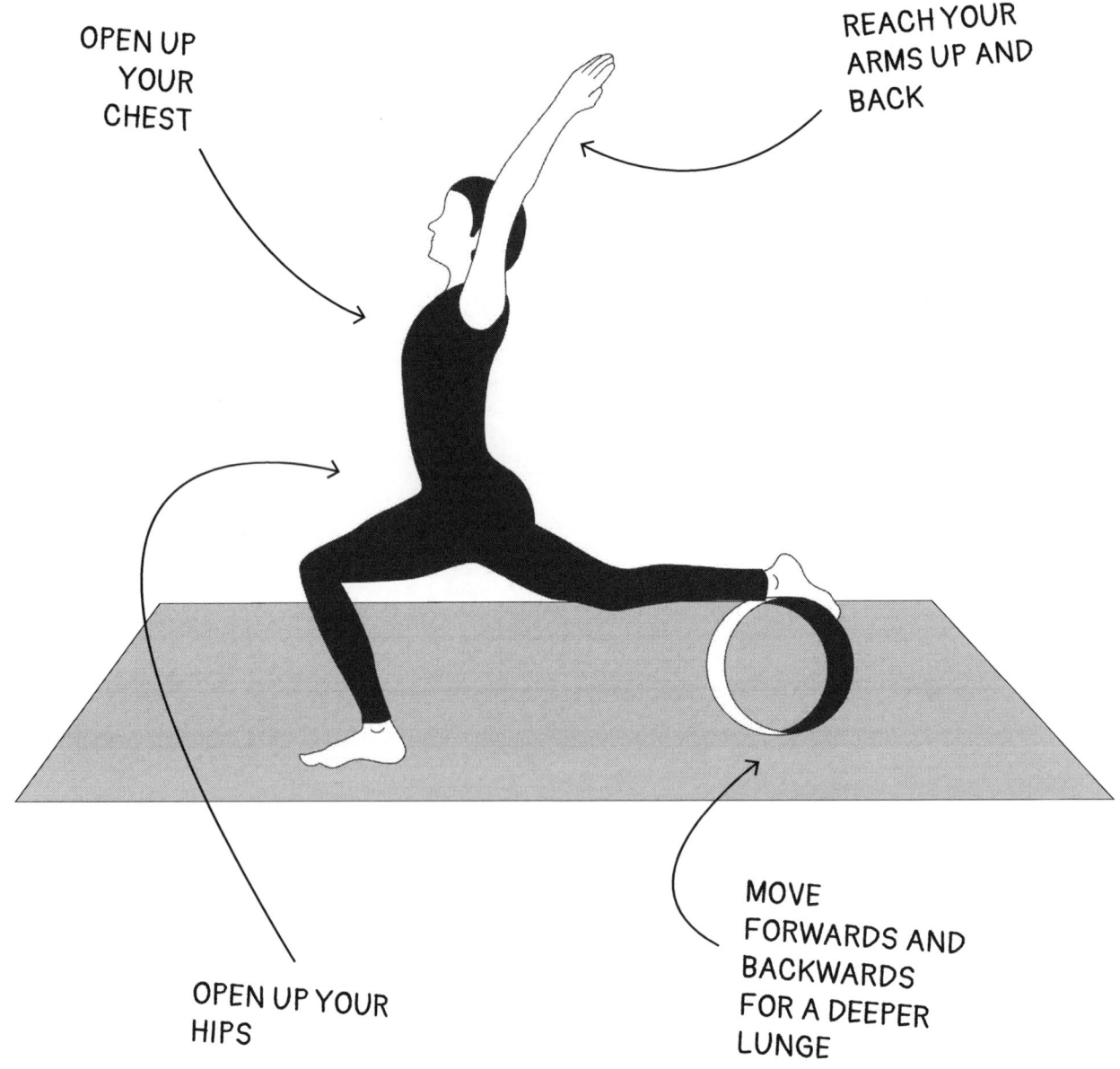

Rolling High Lunge

Anjaneyasana

The Rolling High Lunge stretches both the hamstrings and hips, while also challenging your balance. It can become a dynamic stretch, by rolling the wheel forwards and backwards as you move deeper into the lunge.

1. Start in a standing position, with the wheel on the mat behind you.

2. Lift one leg behind you to rest it on the wheel.

3. Step the other leg forward into a high lunge.

4. Lift your arms and lengthen them towards the back of the room to deepen the stretch.

TARGETS: HAMSTRINGS, HIPS, CHEST, BALANCE

YOGA WHEEL BOOK

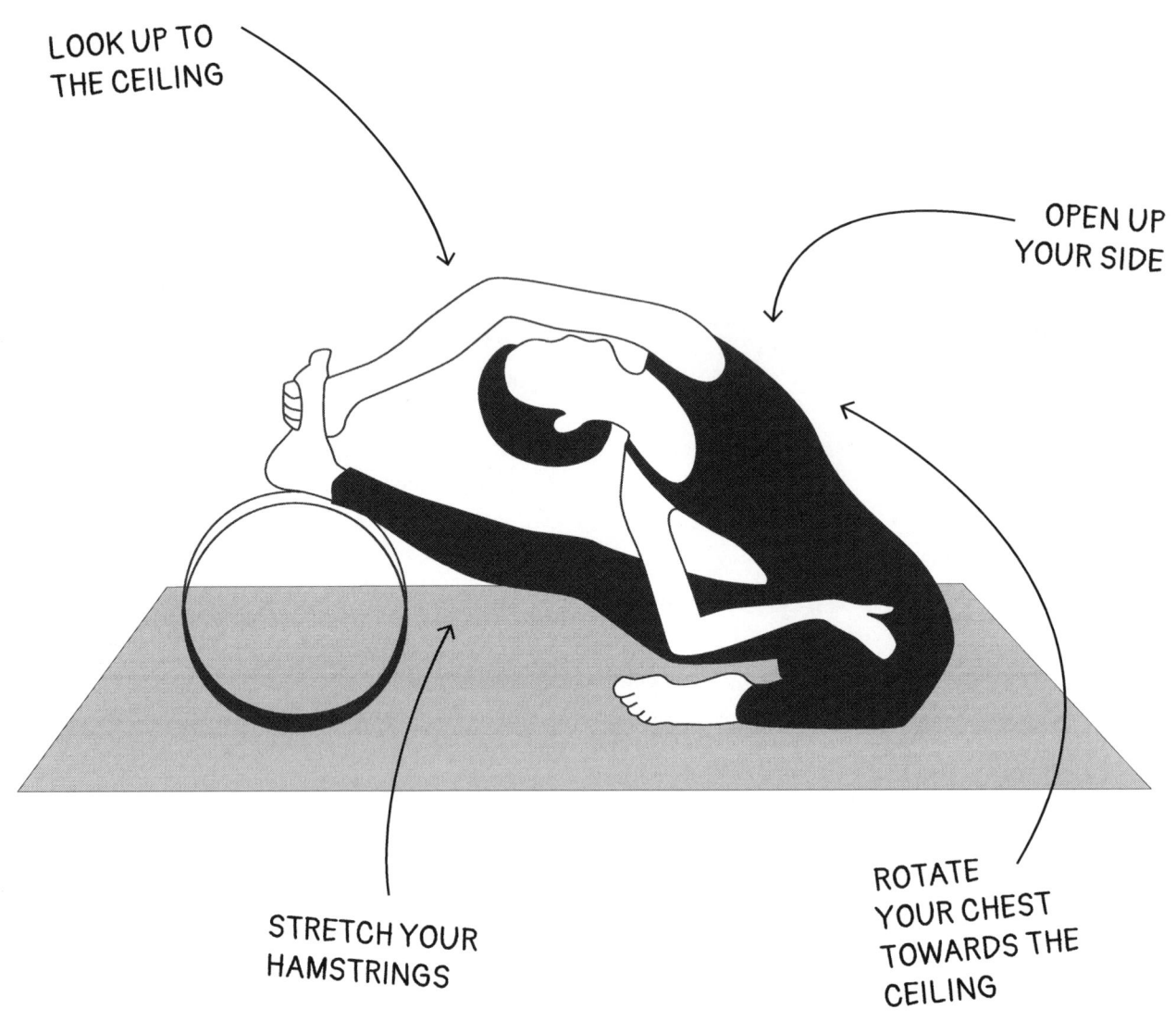

STRETCHES

Revolved Head to Knee

Parvritta Janu Sirshasana

The Revolved Head to Knee is a seated bend that opens up the side, while also twisting the abdominal muscles. Keep the chest open and look upwards for the most effective stretch.

1. Begin in a seated position with your legs extended to the sides.

2. Bend your right knee and bring the sole of your foot towards your left thigh.

3. Slowly lift your left leg to place your heel on the wheel.

4. Extend your right arm to reach the inside of your left foot, as you rotate your chest towards the ceiling.

TARGETS: SPINE, SHOULDERS, SIDE, HAMSTRINGS

YOGA WHEEL BOOK

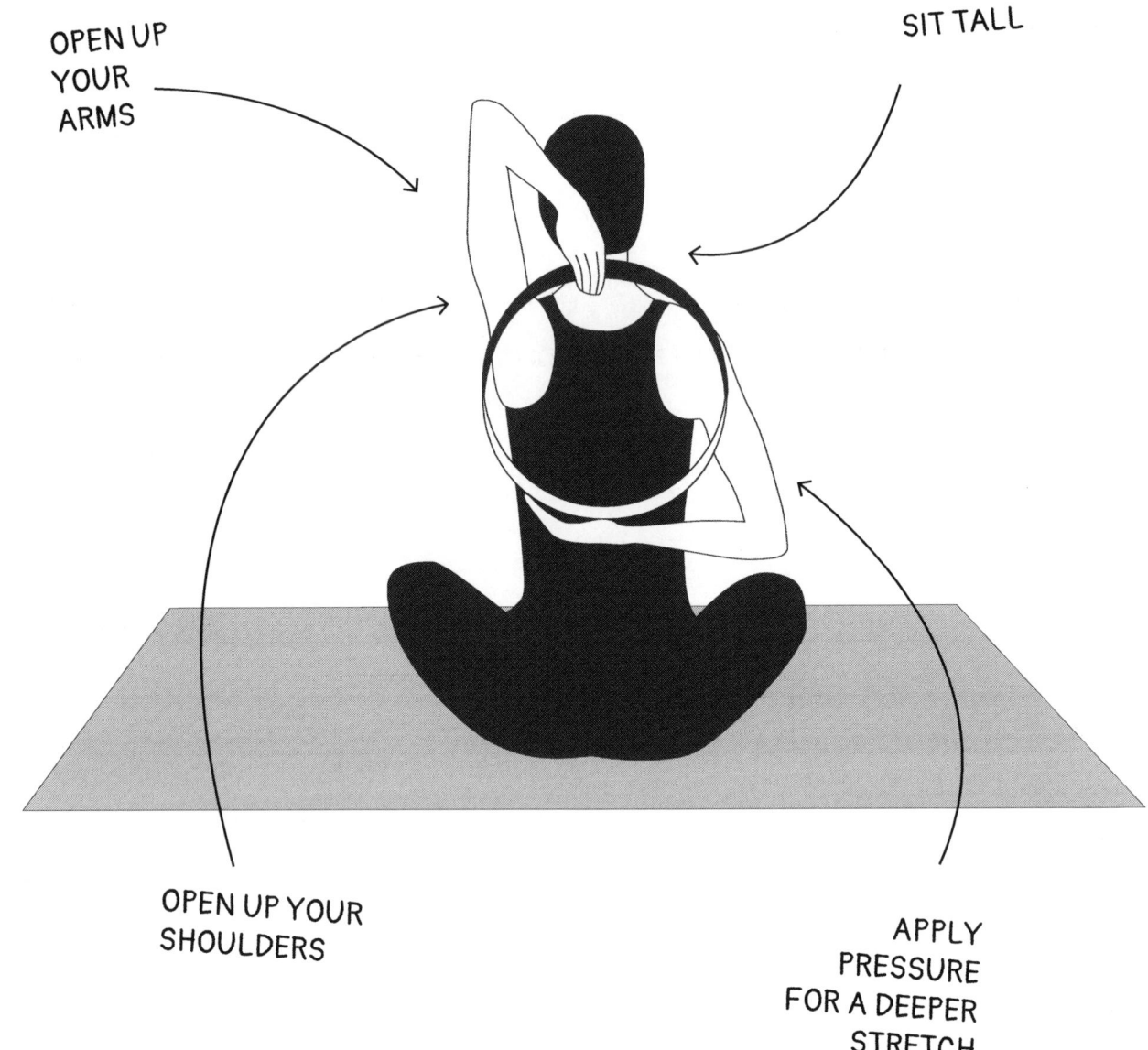

Cow Face

Gomukhasana

The Cow Face is a warm-up stretch that opens up the shoulders and the arms. You can apply pressure on the wheel in this position for a deeper pose.

1. Lift the wheel above your head with one arm, and then bend your elbow to lower it behind your back.

2. Bring your other arm behind your back and rest it on the underside of the wheel.

TARGETS: SHOULDERS, SCAPULA

YOGA WHEEL BOOK

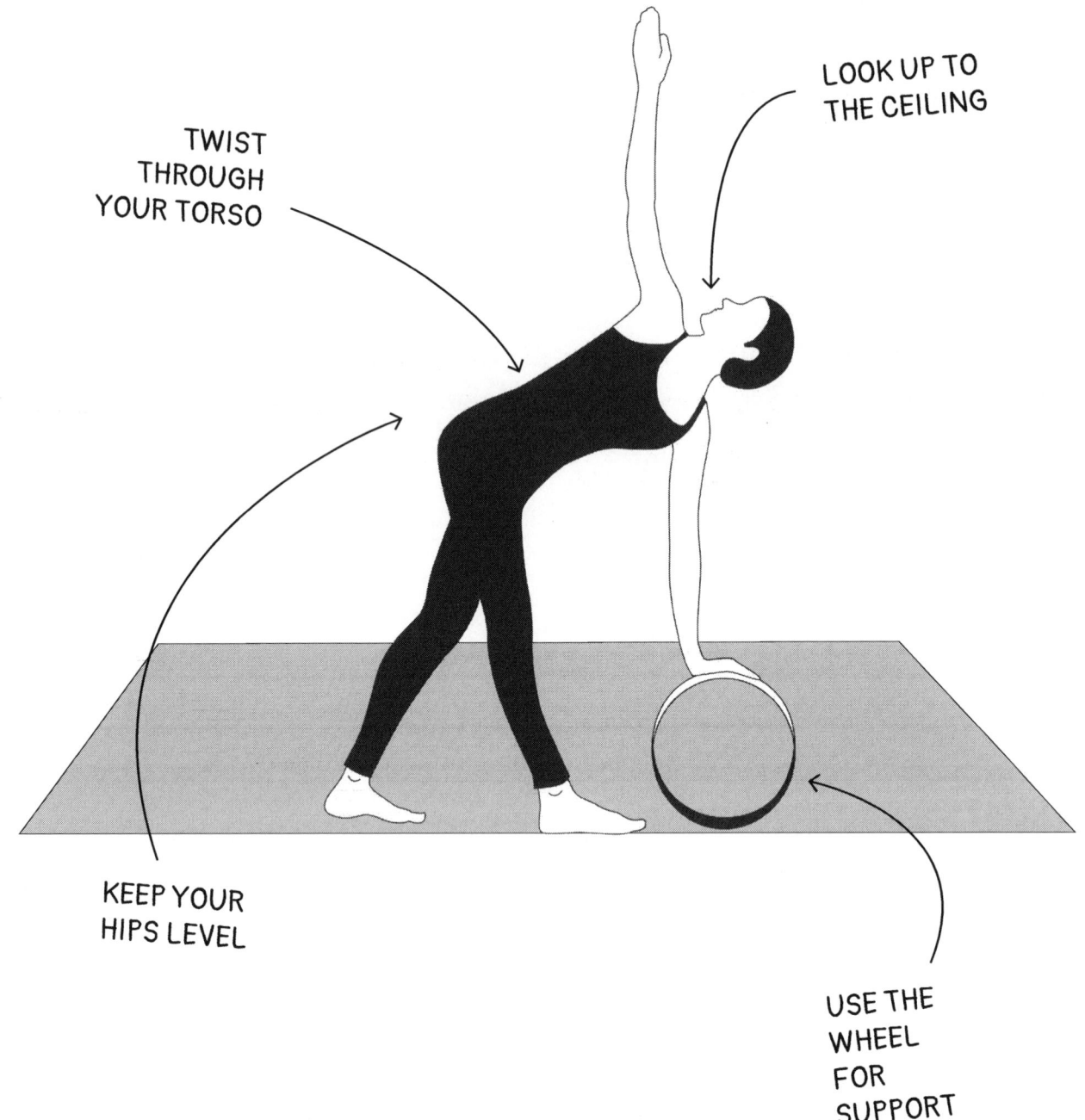

Revolved Forward Fold

Parivrtta Prasarita

The Revolved Forward Fold is a warm-up or cool-down stretch for opening up the chest. Twisting through the torso helps to keep the spine healthy. The wheel acts as a support in this pose as you work towards reaching the floor.

1. Stand with your left foot forward, and the wheel on the mat in front of you.

2. Fold forward from your hips, keeping your torso lengthened.

3. Place your right hand on top of the wheel, and then raise your left hand as you twist your torso towards the ceiling. Keep your hips level and only move from your upper body.

4. Look up to the ceiling as you hold the stretch.

TARGETS: HAMSTRINGS, CALVES, HIPS, BACK, SPINE, SHOULDERS, HIPS

YOGA WHEEL BOOK

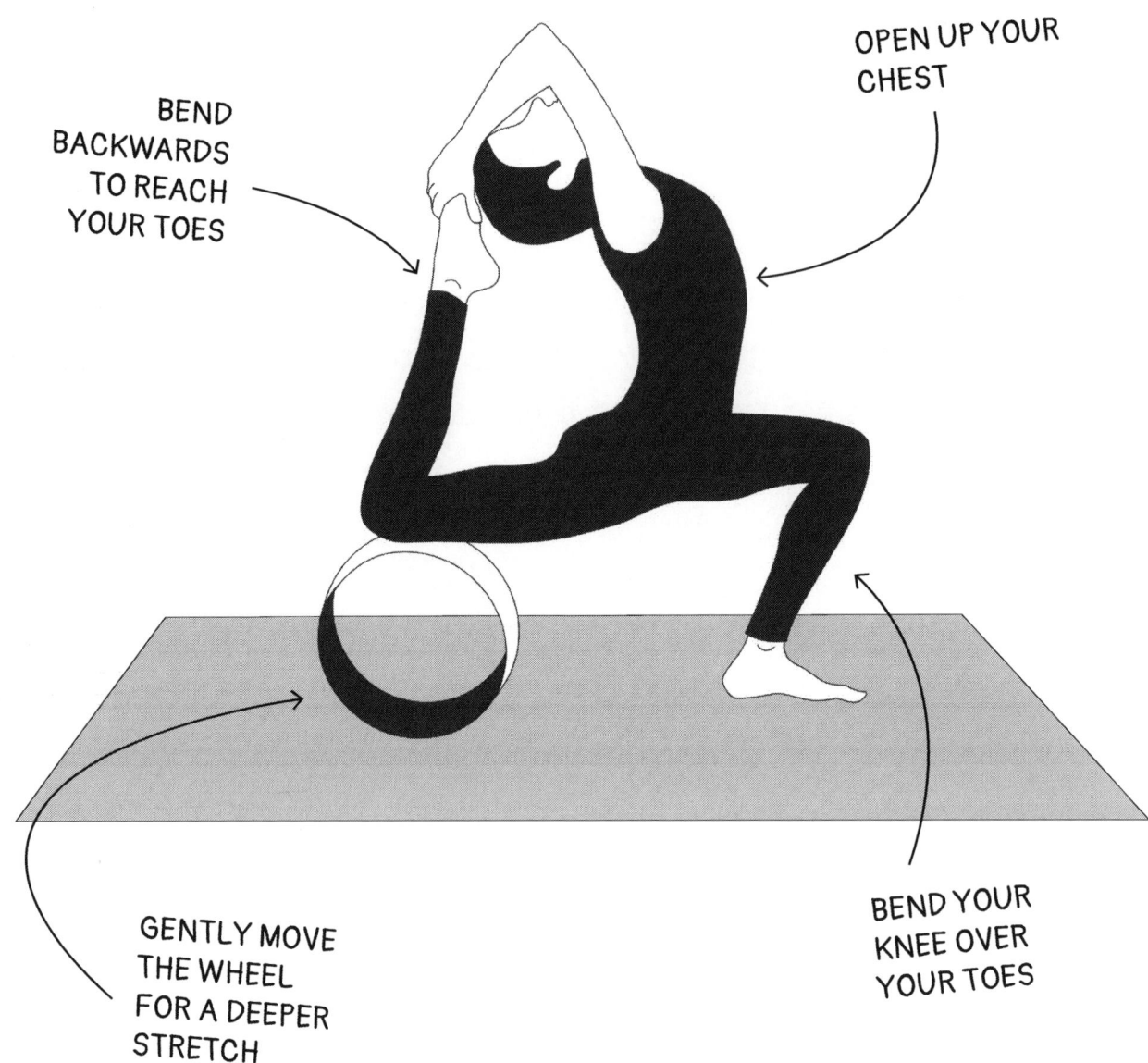

One-Legged King Pigeon

Eka Pada Rajakapotasana

The One-Legged King Pigeon is a hip opener stretch that uses the wheel to assist with a more challenging pose. It can become a dynamic stretch by rolling the wheel gently as you bend backwards.

1. Start in a standing position, with the wheel resting on the mat next to you.

2. Step forward into a deep lunge, so that your front knee is over your toes.

3. Lift your back leg and rest your thigh on the wheel, pointing your toes towards the ceiling.

4. Lift your arms above your head and slowly bend backwards to reach your toes.

TARGETS: BACK, CORE, HIPS, PELVIS, QUADS

YOGA WHEEL BOOK

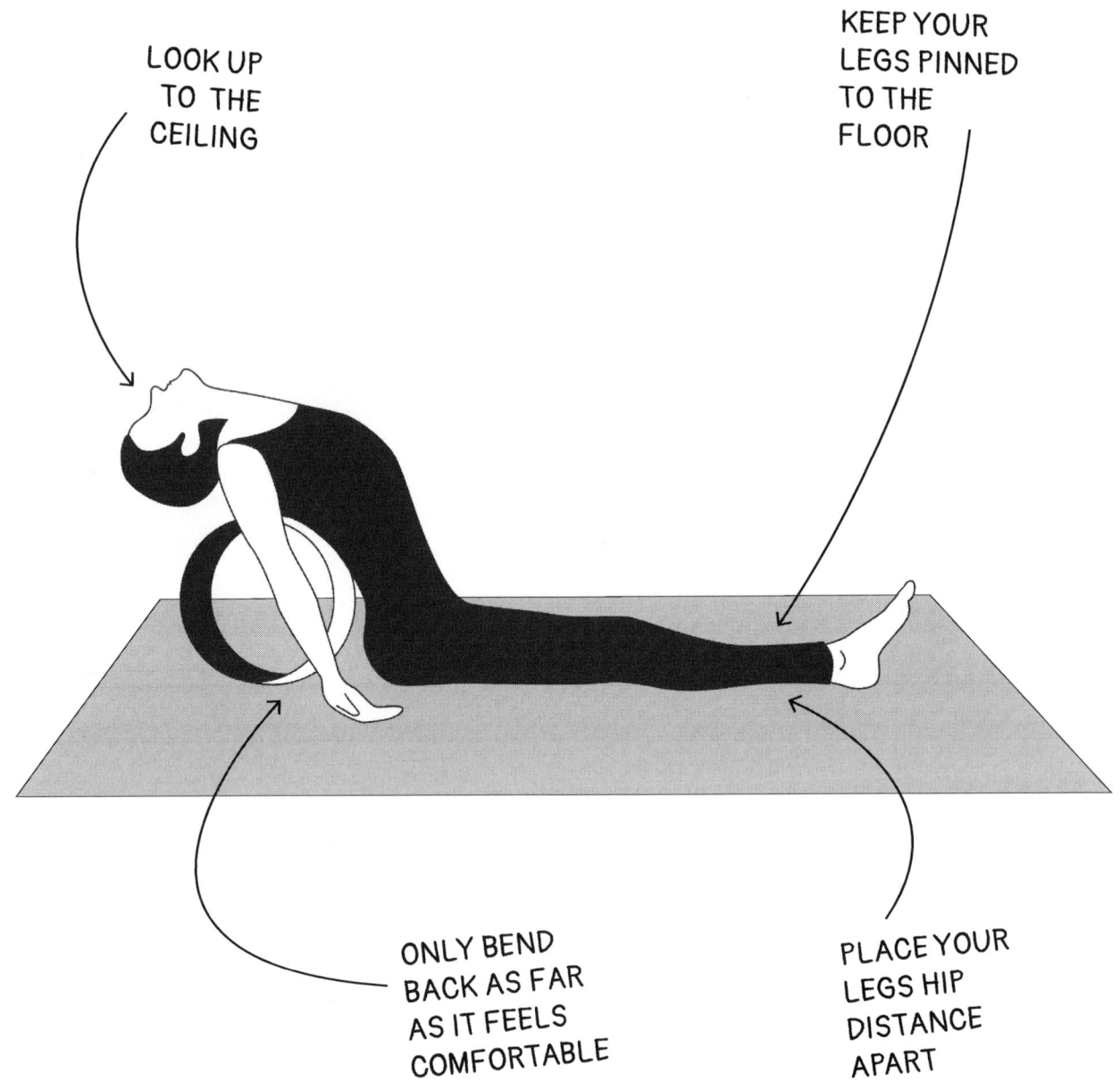

Fish Prep

Matsyasana Prep

This Fish Prep uses the wheel to help you prepare for a full backbend. The backbend is the best way to stretch out a forward hunched spine that comes from sitting at a desk all day or texting.

1. Start sitting on the mat, with the wheel behind you in the centre of your spine.

2. Stretch out your legs, keeping them hip-distance apart and slowly bend backwards.

3. Slowly fold your spine around the wheel, only as far as feels comfortable.

4. Keep your legs pinned to the floor, and look up to the ceiling as you stretch your toes.

TARGETS: POSTURE, BACK, CHEST

YOGA WHEEL BOOK

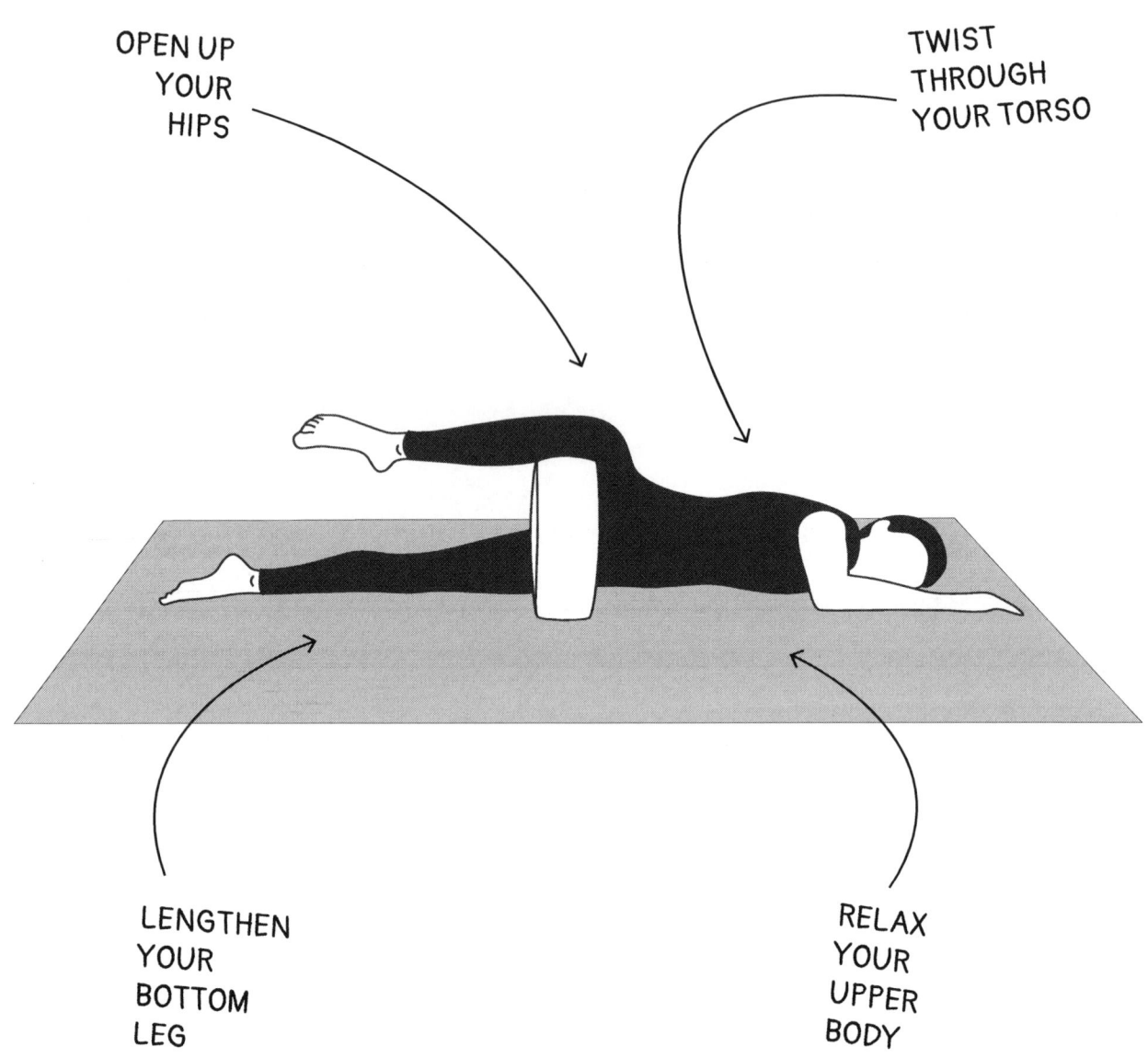

Side-lying Fetal Hip Opener

Parsva Savasana

The Side-lying Fetal Hip Opener is a cool-down position that allows the body to relax and unwind. Using the wheel in this position opens up and stretches the hips.

1. Lie on your left side with the wheel in front of your hips.
2. Bring your right arm over to rest on the floor.
3. Lift your right leg and bring it forward to rest on the wheel.

TARGETS: HIPS

YOGA WHEEL BOOK

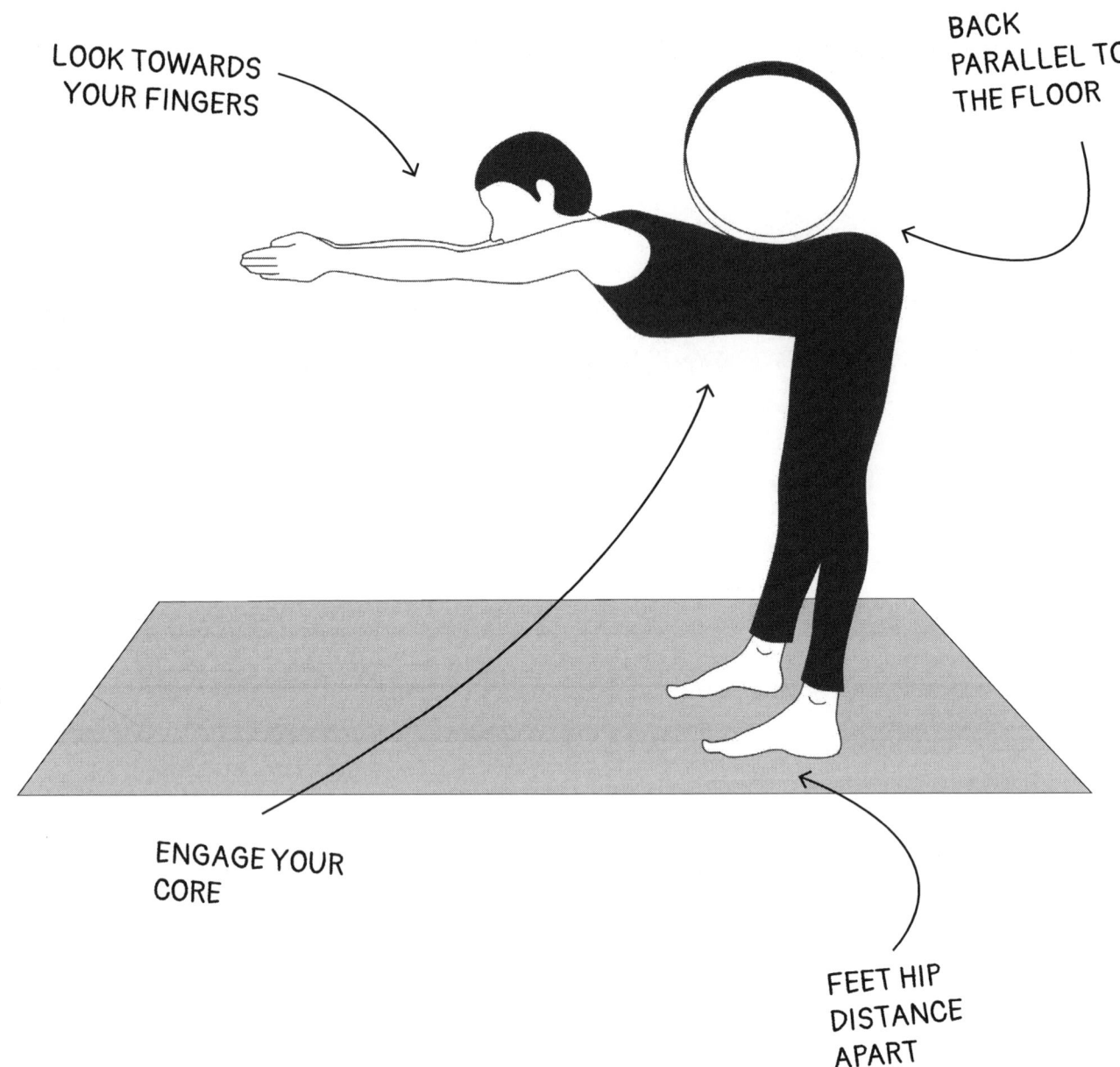

Half Standing Forward Fold

Ardha Uttanasana

The Half Standing Forward Fold is a foundation pose that helps to strengthen the back and improve posture. Balancing the wheel on the back emphasises the need for stability.

1. With the wheel in your hands, bend over to touch the floor.

2. Slowly come back up so that your back is flat and parallel with the floor.

3. Carefully lift the wheel over your head and place it on your back, keeping your core strong.

4. Stretch your arms back out in front of you, then point your fingers away from your body and look forward.

TARGETS: BACK, POSTURE

YOGA WHEEL BOOK

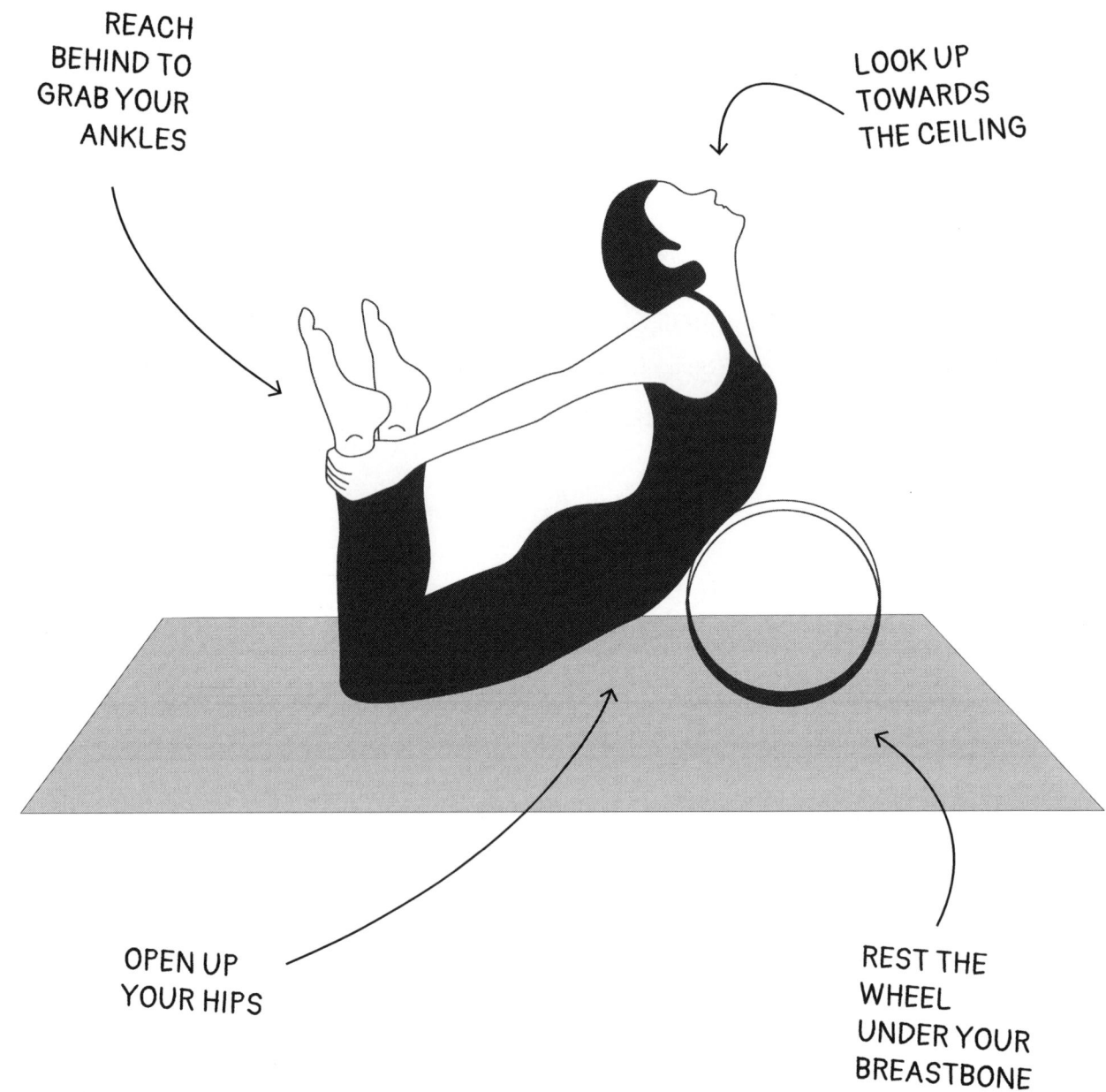

Supported Bow

Dhanurasana

The Supported Bow is a variation of the classic Bow, using the wheel to help you get into a deeper back-bend. This position strengthens the upper back muscles while opening up the shoulders, chest and hip flexors.

1. Start in a full Cobra, with your wrists underneath your shoulders and your shoulders back.

2. Place the wheel in front of you.

3. Slowly lift your feet towards your bottom, and then rest the wheel directly underneath your breastbone.

4. Reach behind and grab your ankles as you look up to the ceiling.

TARGETS: UPPER BACK, CHEST, SHOULDERS, HIP FLEXORS

YOGA WHEEL BOOK

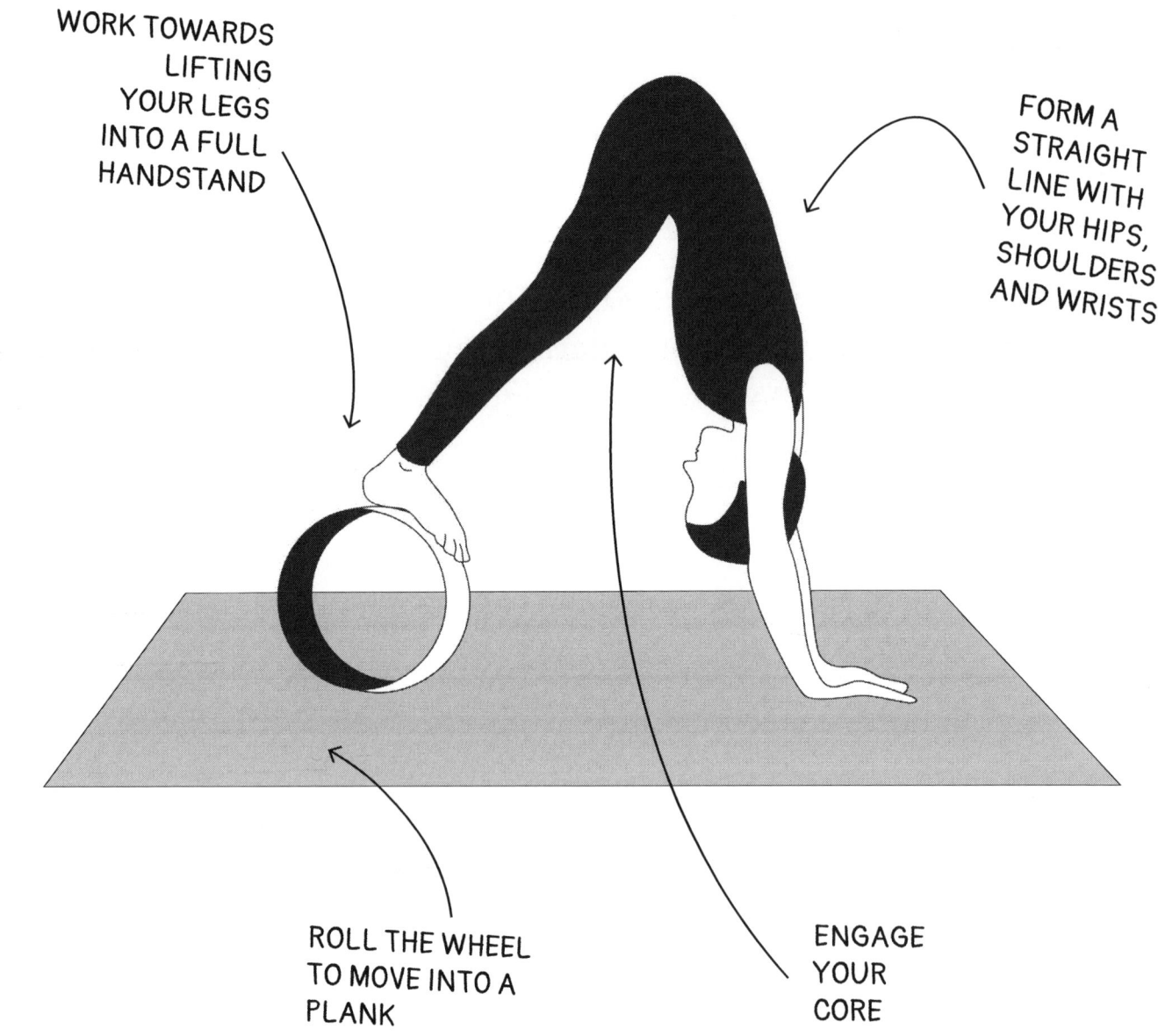

Handstand Prep

Adho Mukha Vrksasana Prep

This Handstand Prep uses the wheel to build confidence and work towards a full handstand position. It will also help familiarise the body with stacking the hips on top of the shoulders and the wrists in one straight line.

1. Start on all fours, with the wheel behind your feet.

2. Engage your core and lift your legs to rest on the wheel in a plank position.

3. Lift your bottom to the ceiling into a pike position. Keep your legs straight as the wheel moves from your shins to your feet.

4. Turn your feet so that they are flat on the wheel.

5. From here you can continue to move between the plank and pike positions, or work towards lifting your legs off the wheel into a full handstand.

TARGETS: SHOULDERS, CORE, STABILITY, SPINE

YOGA WHEEL BOOK

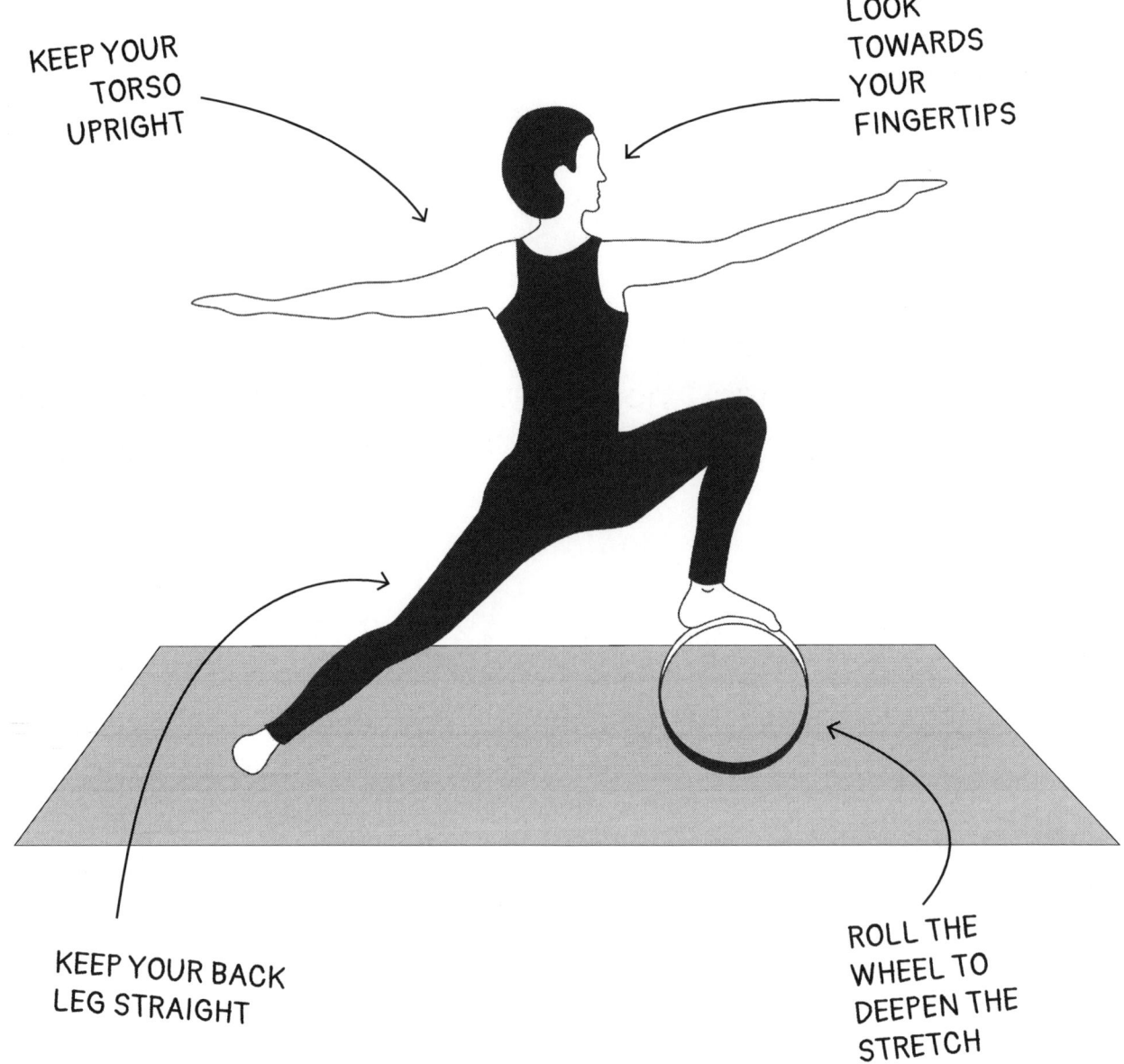

Warrior

Upavistha Virabhadrasana

The Warrior provides a deep stretch to your lower body, whilst also strengthening your arms and legs. Using the wheel in this position allows you to challenge your stability and deepen the pose. It is also possible to make this into a dynamic pose by gently rolling the wheel forwards and backwards.

1. Start standing with your feet hips distance apart, and the wheel on the mat next to you.

2. Step your legs wide, and then lift your right foot onto the wheel.

3. Keep your left leg straight and bend your right knee over your toes.

4. With your torso upright, lift your arms out to the side as you look towards your fingertips.

TARGETS: GLUTES, QUADS, HAMSTRINGS, OBLIQUES, SPINE, CHEST, HIPS, SHOULDERS

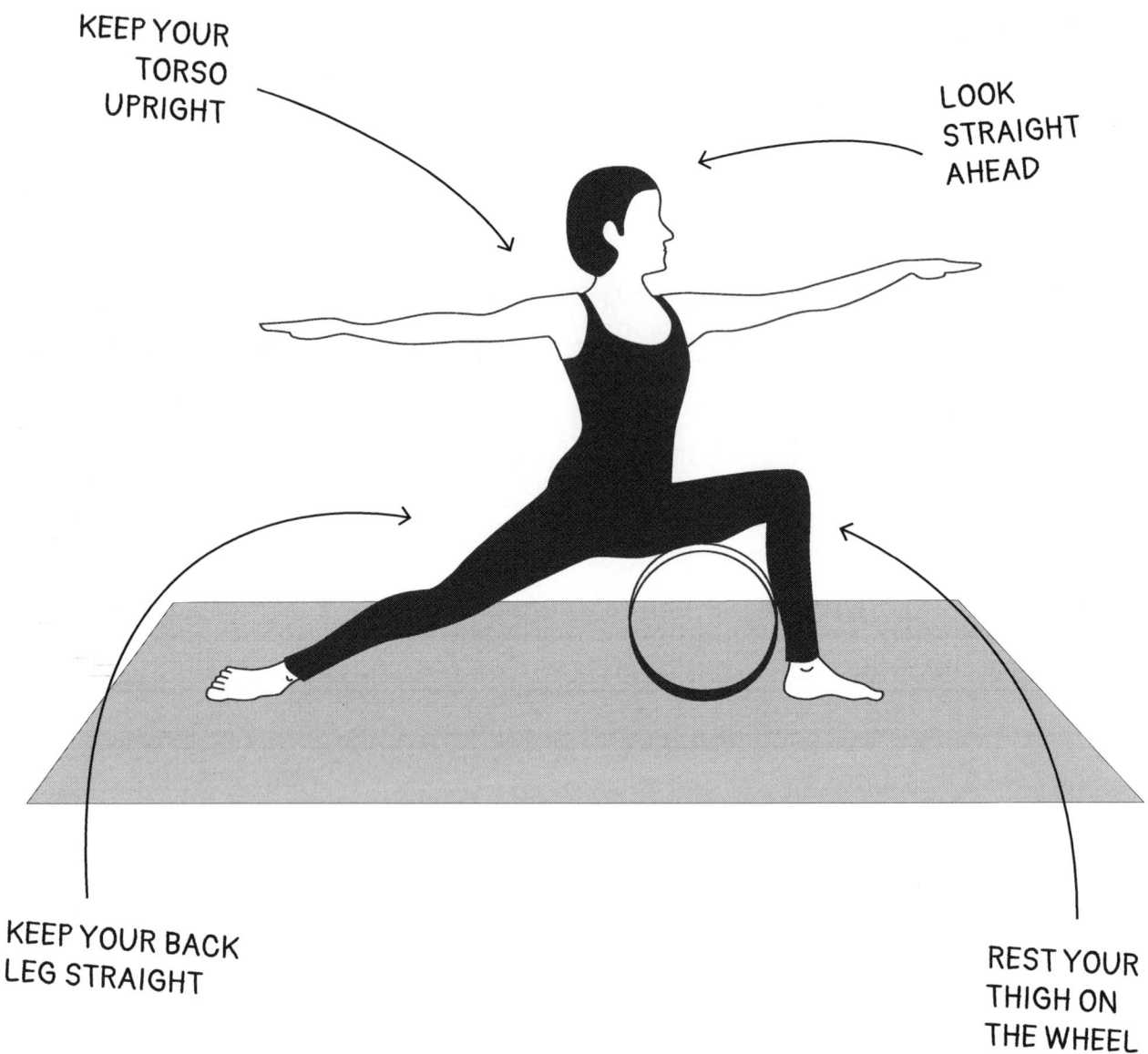

BEGINNER

Seated Warrior

Virabhadrasana

Using the wheel for the Seated Warrior can provide extra stability. With the wheel, you can practice a deeper full-body stretch whilst building up the confidence to attempt more advanced poses.

1. Start in a standing position, with the wheel on the mat in front of you.

2. Step forward into a lunge with your right leg, and then rest your thigh on the wheel.

3. Step your left leg back and straighten it as you move deeper into the lunge.

4. Lift your arms out to the side as you gaze forward.

TARGETS: UPPER BACK, HAMSTRINGS, HIPS

YOGA WHEEL BOOK

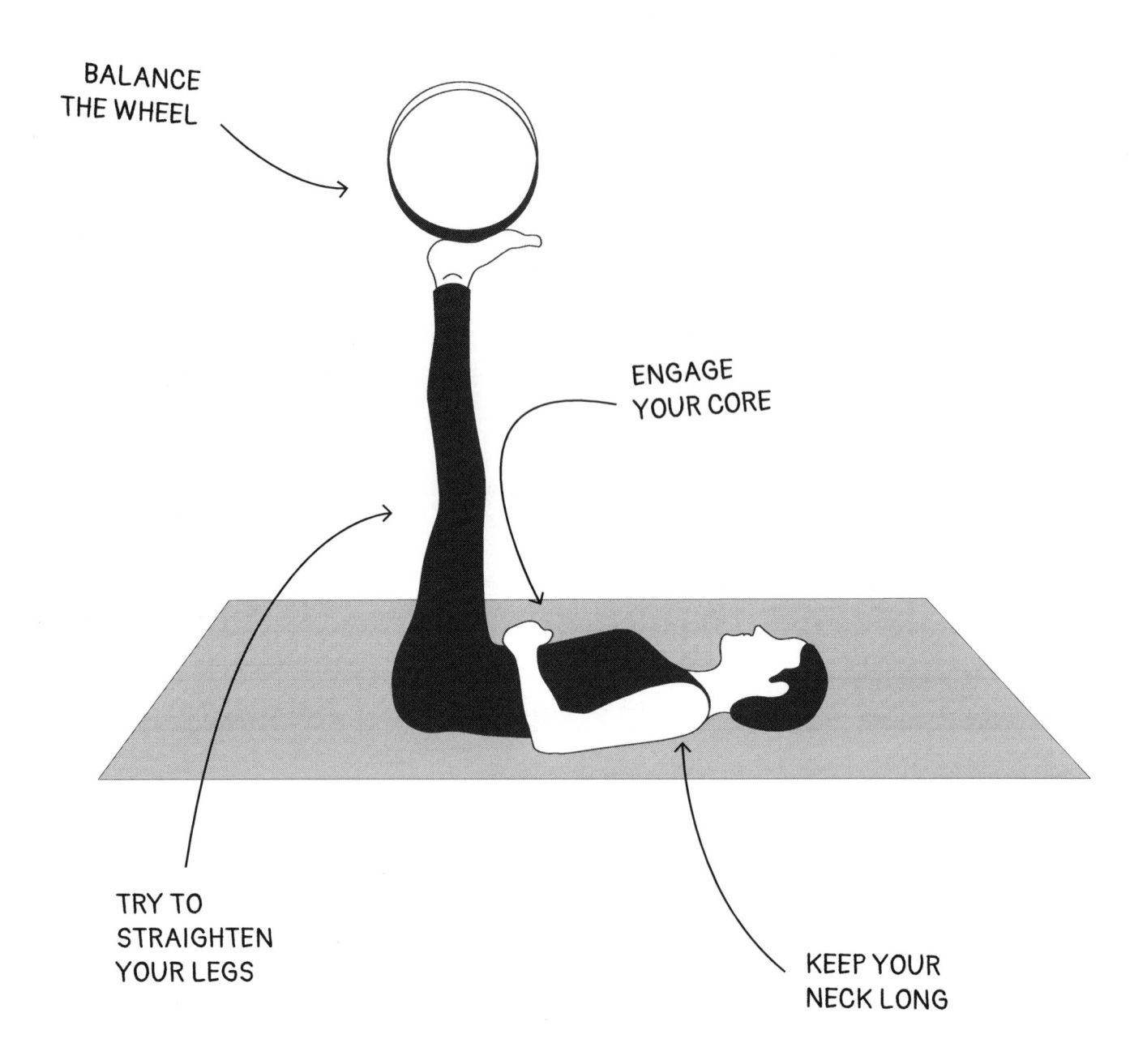

BALANCE THE WHEEL

ENGAGE YOUR CORE

TRY TO STRAIGHTEN YOUR LEGS

KEEP YOUR NECK LONG

Double Leg Raise

Uttana Padasana

The Double Leg Raise is a great way to strengthen the abs. The balance with the wheel forces slower and more careful movement, using core strength for stability.

1. Start lying on your back, with your hands by your side and your feet together.

2. With your pelvis in neutral, bend your knees towards your chest and balance the wheel on your feet.

3. Extend your legs upwards as you balance the wheel on your feet.

4. For an added challenge, lower your legs slightly to work your core. Try not to drop the wheel!

TARGETS: UPPER BACK, HAMSTRINGS, HIPS

YOGA WHEEL BOOK

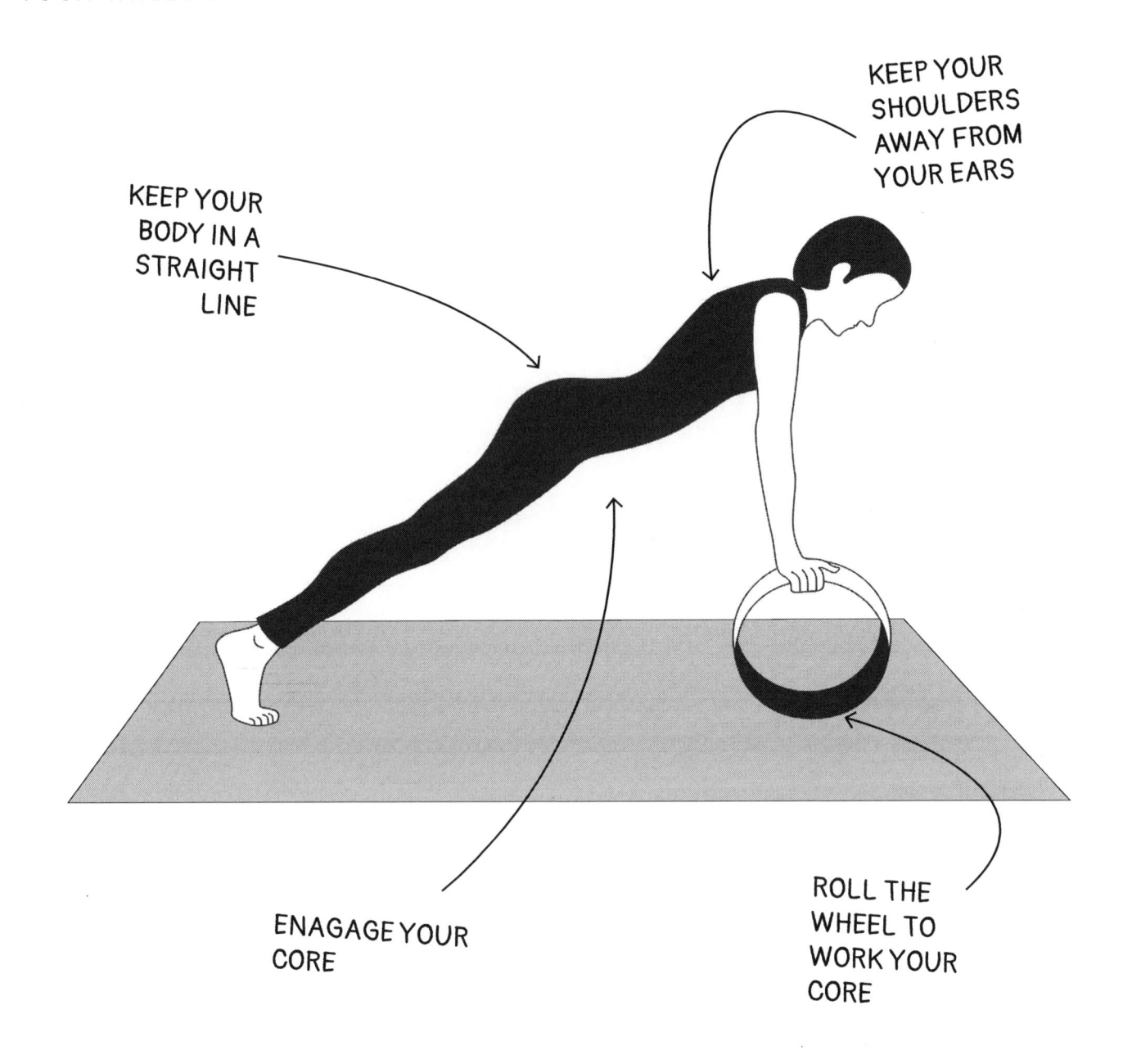

KEEP YOUR SHOULDERS AWAY FROM YOUR EARS

KEEP YOUR BODY IN A STRAIGHT LINE

ENAGAGE YOUR CORE

ROLL THE WHEEL TO WORK YOUR CORE

High Plank

Phalakasana

The High Plank uses the wheel to improve strength and balance. You can also move the wheel forwards and backwards to work the core.

1. Start in a standing position, with the wheel on the mat in front of you.

2. Bend your knees and reach down to put your hands on the wheel.

3. As you press down on the wheel, step your feet back into the High Plank.

4. Bring your shoulders away from your ears and engage your core.

5. For an extra challenge, move the wheel in a tiny forward and backwards motion. Move from the shoulders and keep your body straight.

TARGETS: CORE, BALANCE, ARMS, SHOULDERS

YOGA WHEEL BOOK

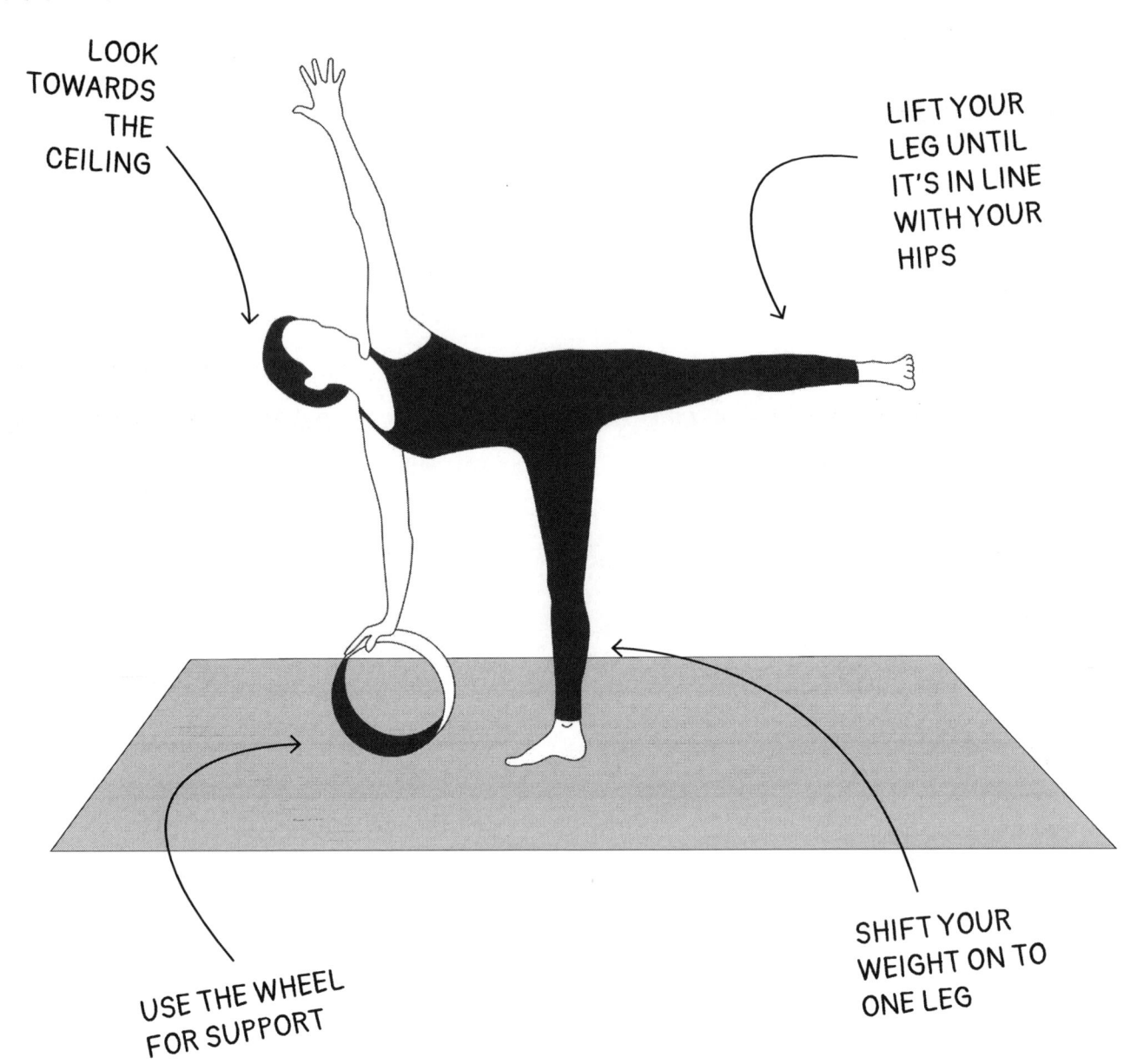

LOOK TOWARDS THE CEILING

LIFT YOUR LEG UNTIL IT'S IN LINE WITH YOUR HIPS

USE THE WHEEL FOR SUPPORT

SHIFT YOUR WEIGHT ON TO ONE LEG

Half Moon

Ardha Chandrasana

The Half Moon works on challenging your balance and strength. The wheel acts as a support, elevating your hand off the floor and helping with alignment.

1. Start in a warrior pose and place the wheel on the mat, in front of your right foot.

2. Reach your right arm towards the wheel, and shift your weight onto your right leg.

3. Float your left leg up until its in line with your hips.

4. Reach your left hand to the ceiling, open up your chest and look upwards.

TARGETS: BALANCE, CORE

YOGA WHEEL BOOK

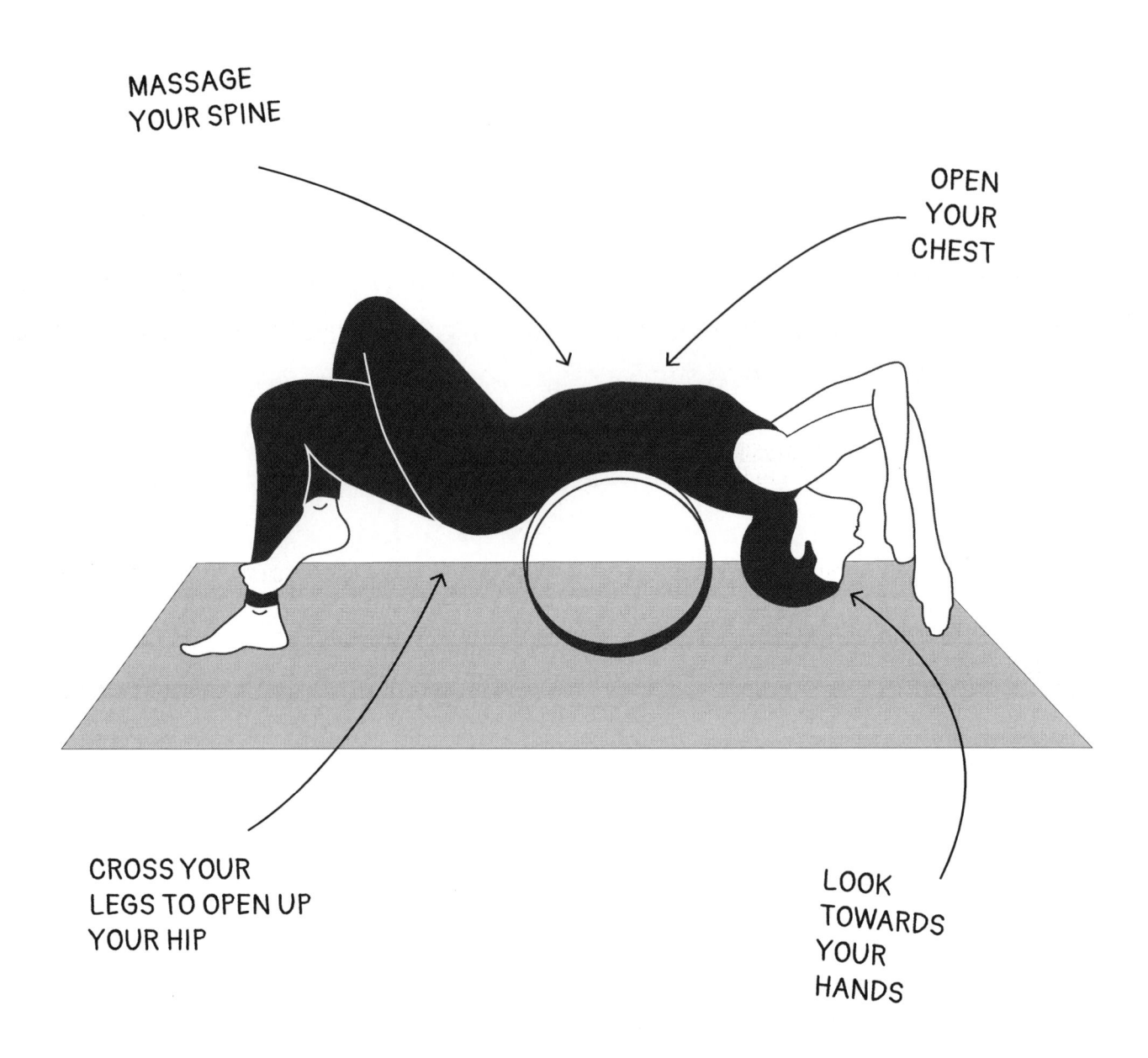

MASSAGE YOUR SPINE

OPEN YOUR CHEST

CROSS YOUR LEGS TO OPEN UP YOUR HIP

LOOK TOWARDS YOUR HANDS

Lotus Fish

Padma Matsyasana

The Lotus Fish uses the wheel to make backbends more accessible. This cross-legged position allows you to start working towards the full backbend pose while also stretching out the hips.

1. Start in a seated position with your hands behind your head and your lower back resting on the wheel.

2. With your knees bent and your feet flat on the floor, slowly lean back onto the wheel.

3. Bend backwards until the wheel is in the centre of your spine. Then, lift your bottom off the floor and hang your head back over the wheel.

4. Cross your arms in front of your face, and lift one leg over the other.

TARGETS: SPINE, CHEST, HIPS, GLUTES

YOGA WHEEL BOOK

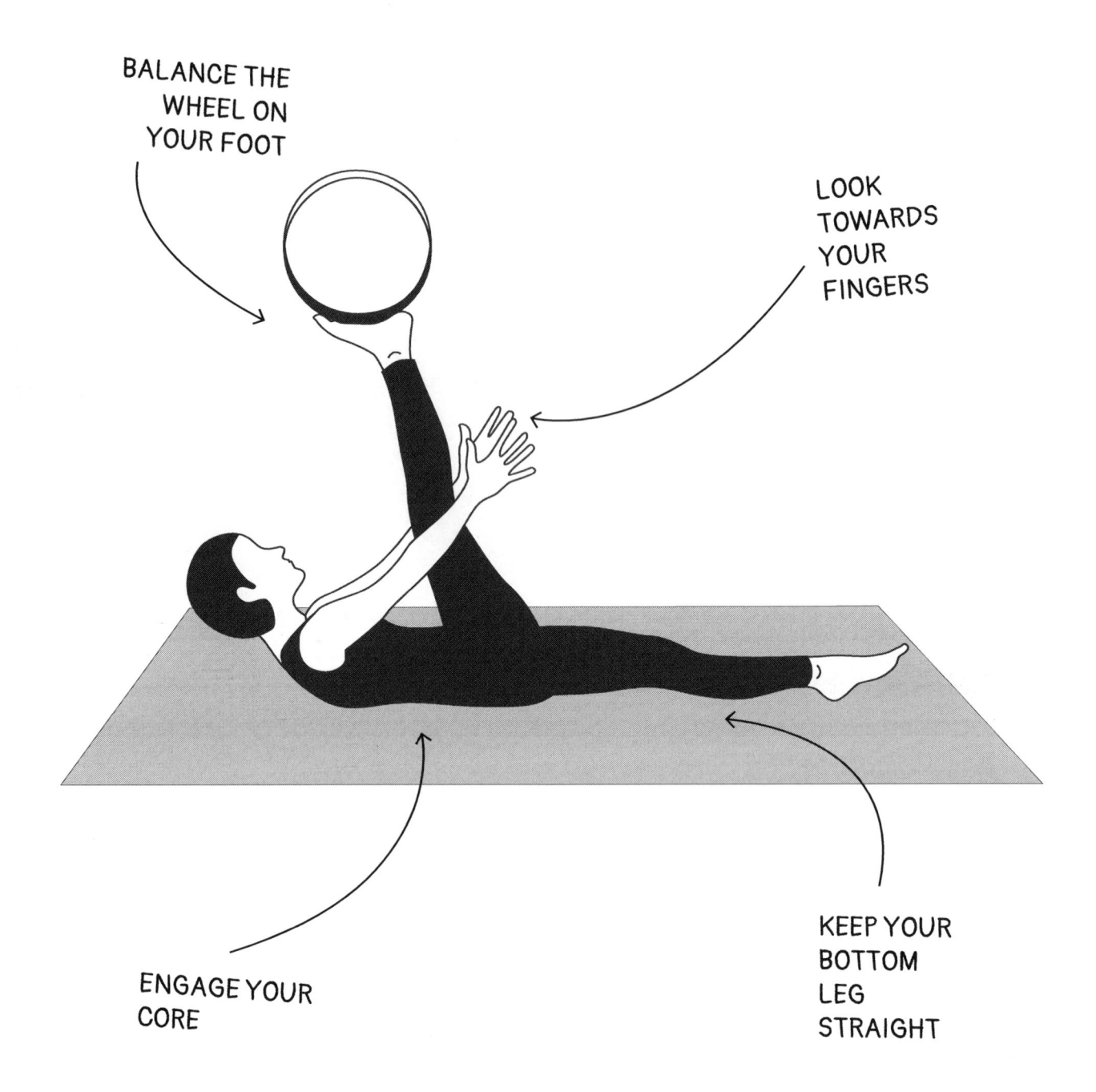

BALANCE THE WHEEL ON YOUR FOOT

LOOK TOWARDS YOUR FINGERS

ENGAGE YOUR CORE

KEEP YOUR BOTTOM LEG STRAIGHT

BEGINNER

One-legged Half Boat

Eka Pada Ardha Navasana

The One-legged Half Boat is perfect for working towards a full Boat pose. It works on core strength and stability. Using the wheel in this position adds an extra challenge of balance and focus.

1. Start by lying on your back with the wheel by your side.

2. Bend your right knee in towards your chest and balance the wheel on the sole of your foot.

3. Extend your right leg up to the ceiling, balancing the wheel. Make sure that the left leg is straight and pointing forwards.

4. With your pelvis in neutral, slowly peel your shoulders off the mat. Reach your arms forwards, past your legs and look towards them.

TARGETS: CORE, STABILITY

YOGA WHEEL BOOK

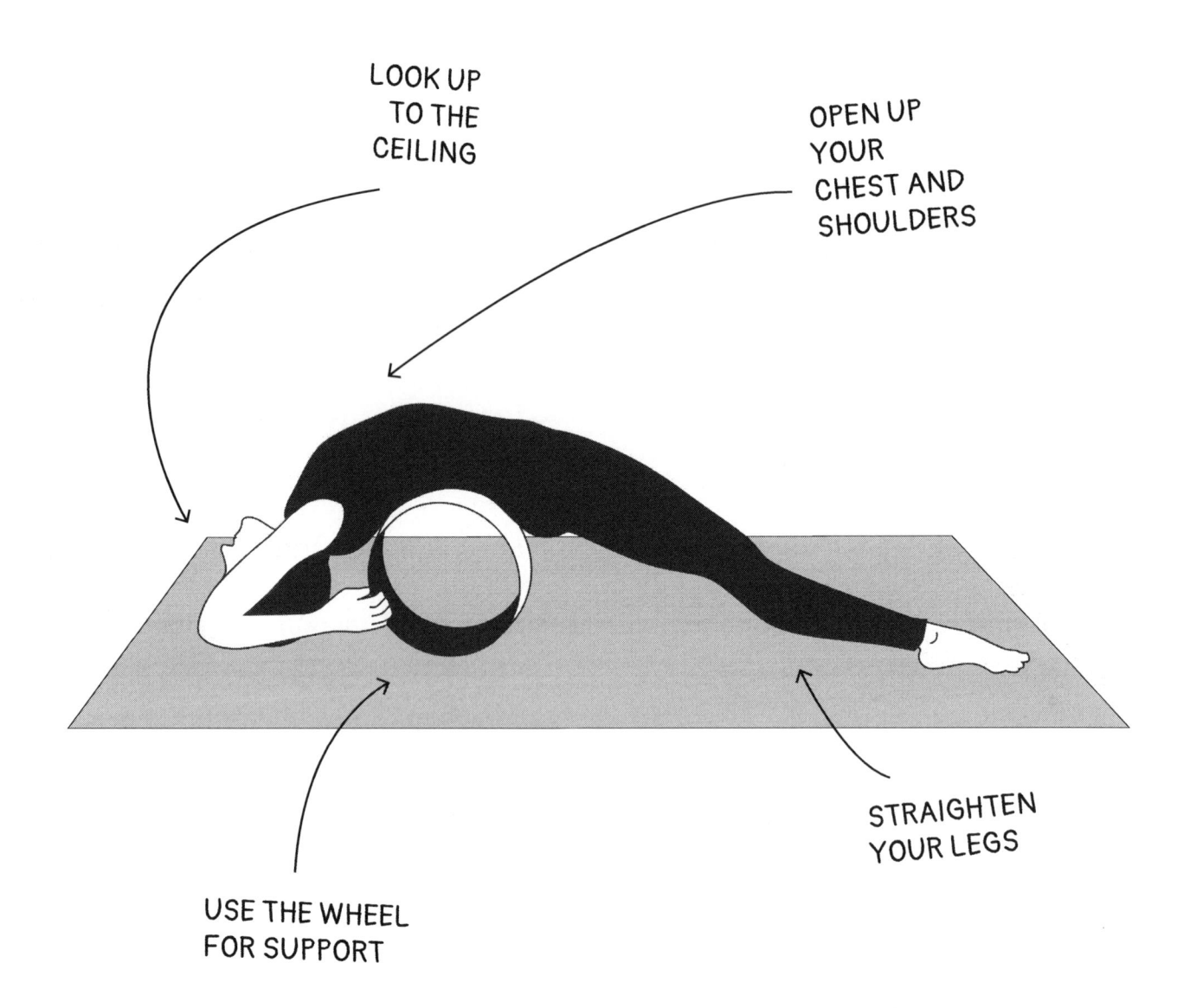

LOOK UP
TO THE
CEILING

OPEN UP
YOUR
CHEST AND
SHOULDERS

USE THE WHEEL
FOR SUPPORT

STRAIGHTEN
YOUR LEGS

INTERMEDIATE

Fish

Urdhva Dhanurasana

The Fish offers a deep stretch for the front of the body, including the chest and shoulders. Using the wheel in this position gives additional support, and also allows a deeper pose.

1. Start sitting on the floor with your legs extended and the wheel in the centre of your back.

2. Lean back and lift your hips to place your spine over the top of the wheel, allowing the wheel to move with your body.

3. Bring your arms above your head until your forearms are flat on the mat, and then grab hold of the wheel.

TARGETS: CHEST, SPINE, HIPS, SHOULDERS

YOGA WHEEL BOOK

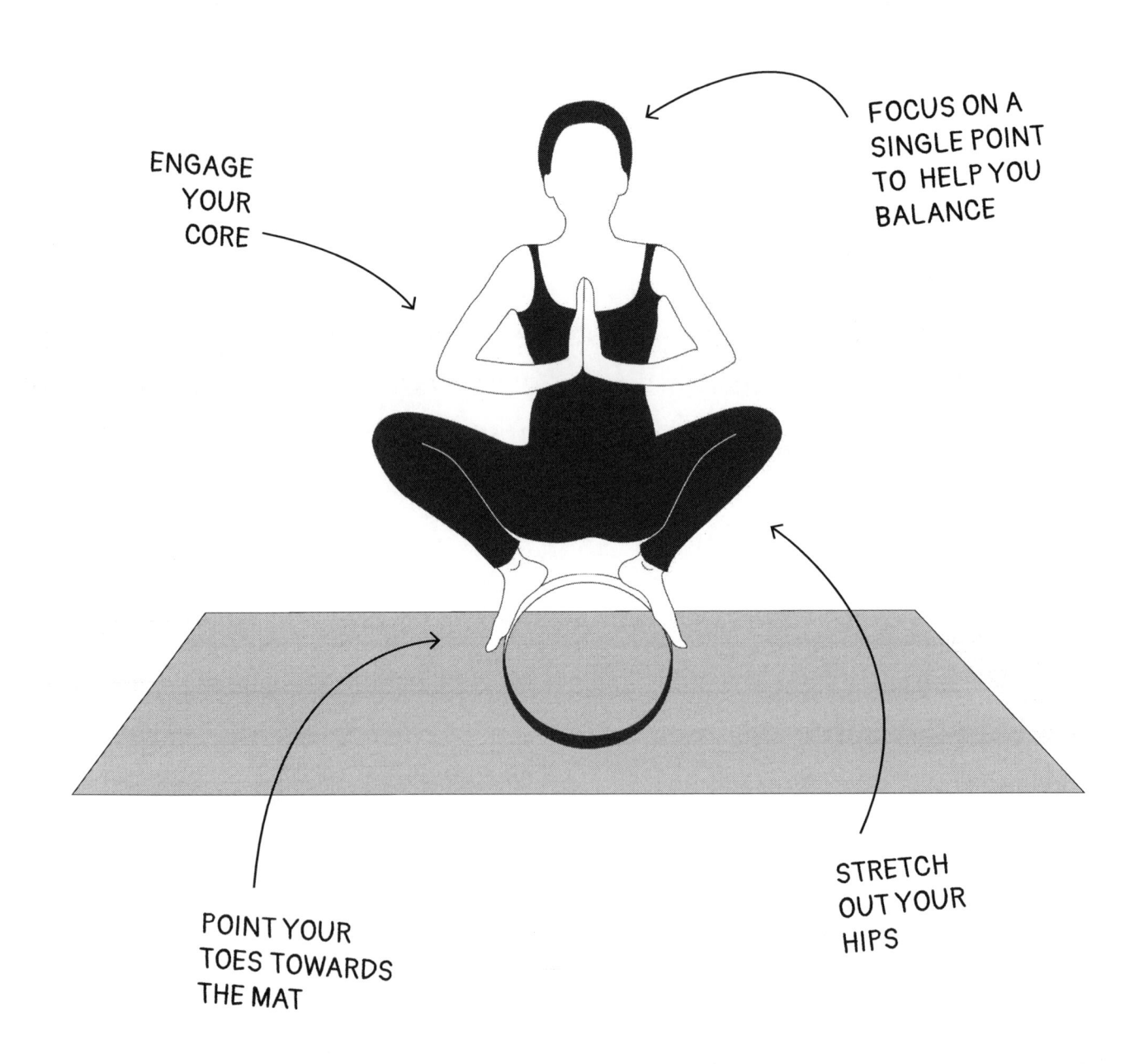

FOCUS ON A SINGLE POINT TO HELP YOU BALANCE

ENGAGE YOUR CORE

STRETCH OUT YOUR HIPS

POINT YOUR TOES TOWARDS THE MAT

INTERMEDIATE

Garland

Malasana

The Garland helps you to practice balance and focus. It is also great for strengthening the pelvis and opening up the hips. Using the wheel to balance in this position forces you to maintain good posture and strengthen your core.

1. Start in a standing position with the wheel in front of you on the mat.

2. Place both hands on the wheel. Bend your right leg and lift your foot onto the wheel, with your toes pointing towards the mat.

3. Once your right leg is in position, bring your left leg onto the wheel and balance in a squat position.

4. Bring your hands into prayer in the centre of your chest.

TARGETS: HIPS, ANKLES, PELVIS, CORE

YOGA WHEEL BOOK

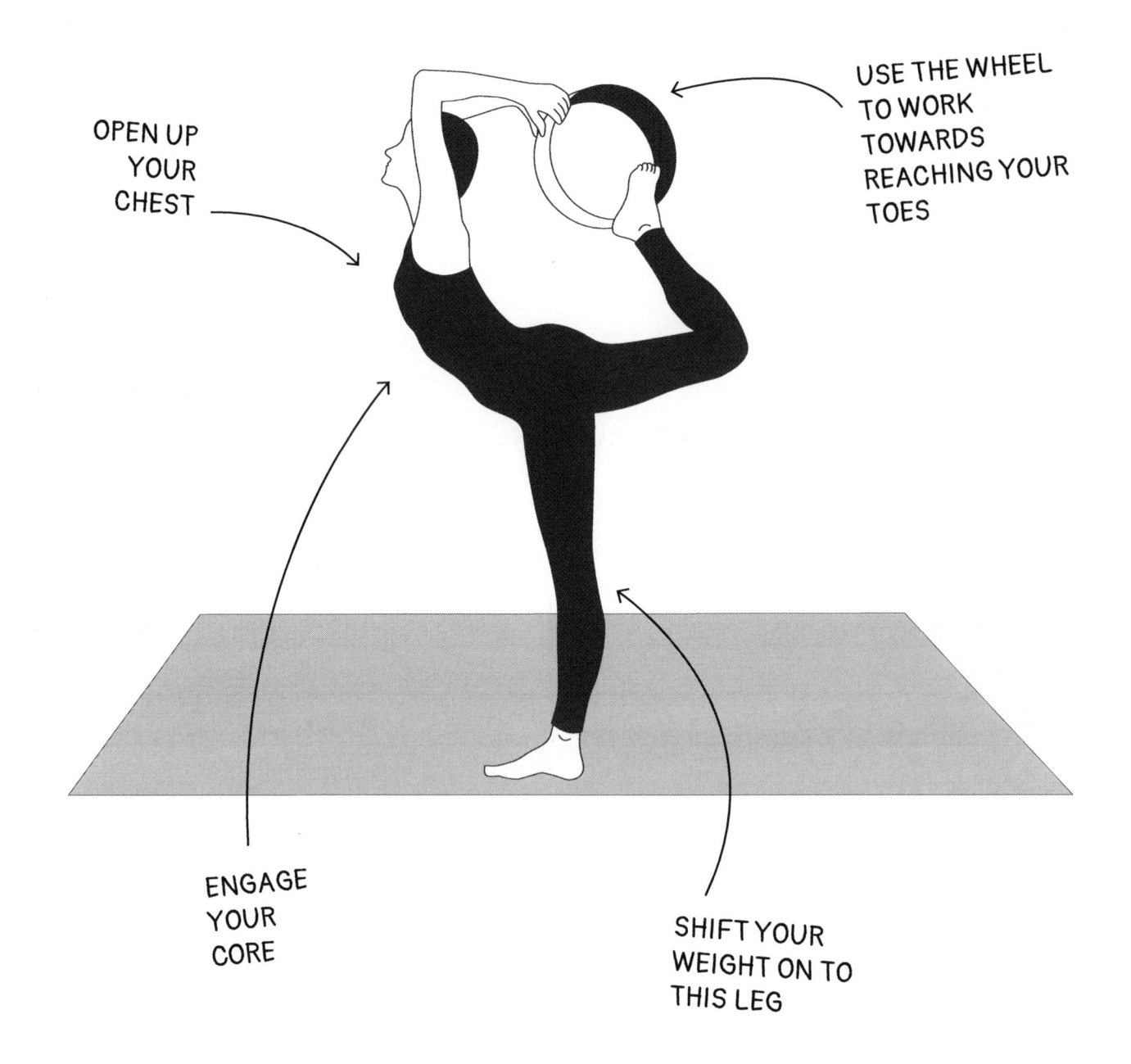

OPEN UP
YOUR
CHEST

USE THE WHEEL
TO WORK
TOWARDS
REACHING YOUR
TOES

ENGAGE
YOUR
CORE

SHIFT YOUR
WEIGHT ON TO
THIS LEG

INTERMEDIATE

Dancer

Natarajasana Hasta

The Dancer opens up the entire front body and is a great way to challenge your balance. Using the wheel in this position helps you achieve the pose even if you can't quite reach your toes yet.

1. Start in a standing position, holding the wheel, with your right palm facing up inside the wheel.

2. Lift your right foot and place it inside the wheel.

3. Gently lift your leg backwards and move the wheel behind you.

4. Rotate your right arm to grip the outside of the wheel, and then bring your left arm over your head to grab the other side of the wheel.

TARGETS: CHEST, SHOULDERS, HIPS, BALANCE

YOGA WHEEL BOOK

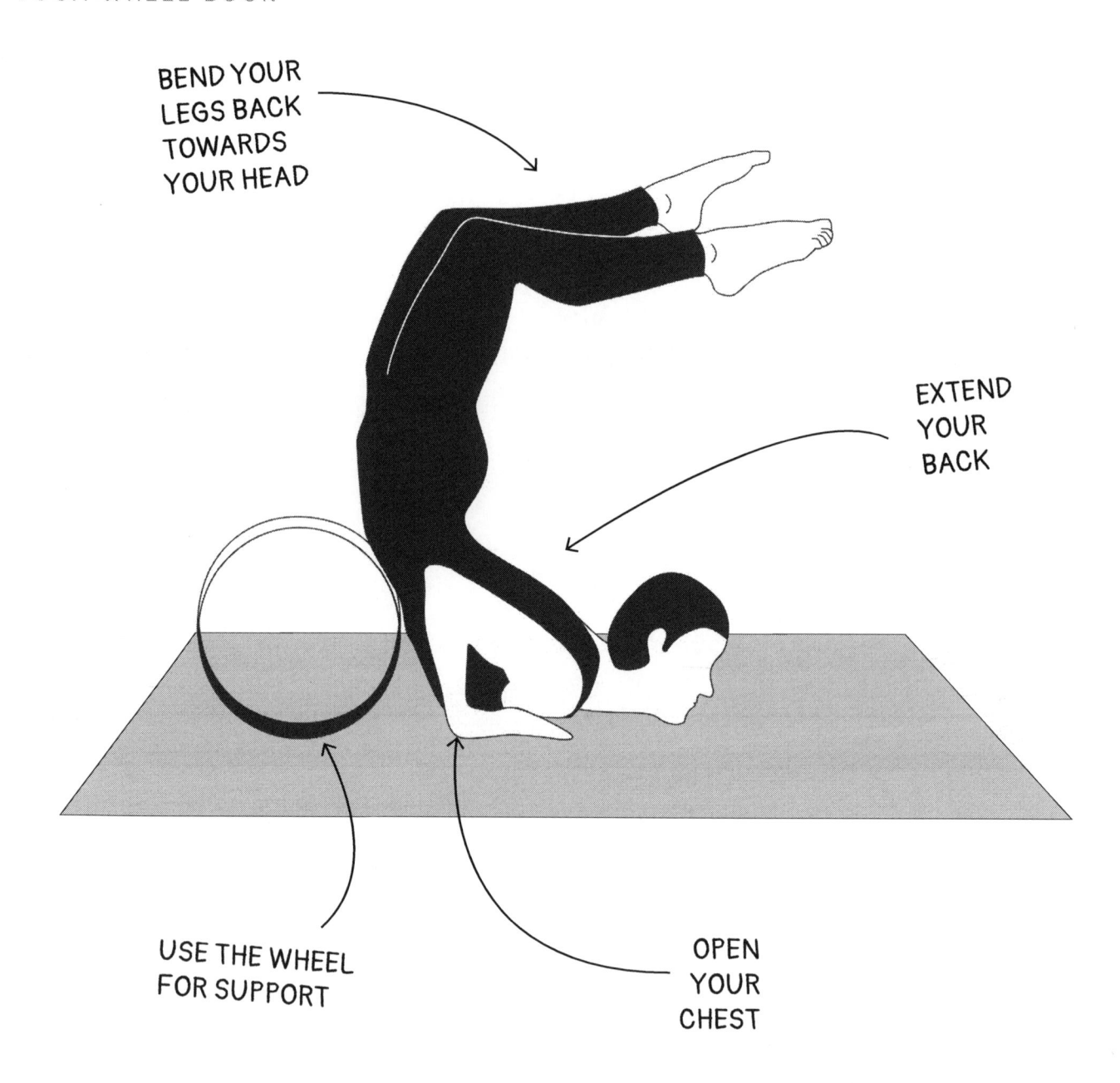

BEND YOUR
LEGS BACK
TOWARDS
YOUR HEAD

EXTEND
YOUR
BACK

USE THE WHEEL
FOR SUPPORT

OPEN
YOUR
CHEST

INTERMEDIATE

Locust

Salabhasana

The Locust can be practiced to prepare for more advanced backbends. It opens up the chest and helps to improve posture. Using the wheel can help you to get into this pose and provide extra support.

1. Start by kneeling on your mat, with the wheel directly in front of you.

2. Bring your hands down to the mat with the wheel underneath your belly.

3. Straighten your legs behind you and then bring your chin to the mat.

4. Reach your hand behind you and grab hold of the wheel.

5. Lift both legs off the mat and bring your feet towards your head.

6. Bring your hands off the wheel so that they are resting on the mat.

TARGETS: CORE, SHOULDERS, BACK

YOGA WHEEL BOOK

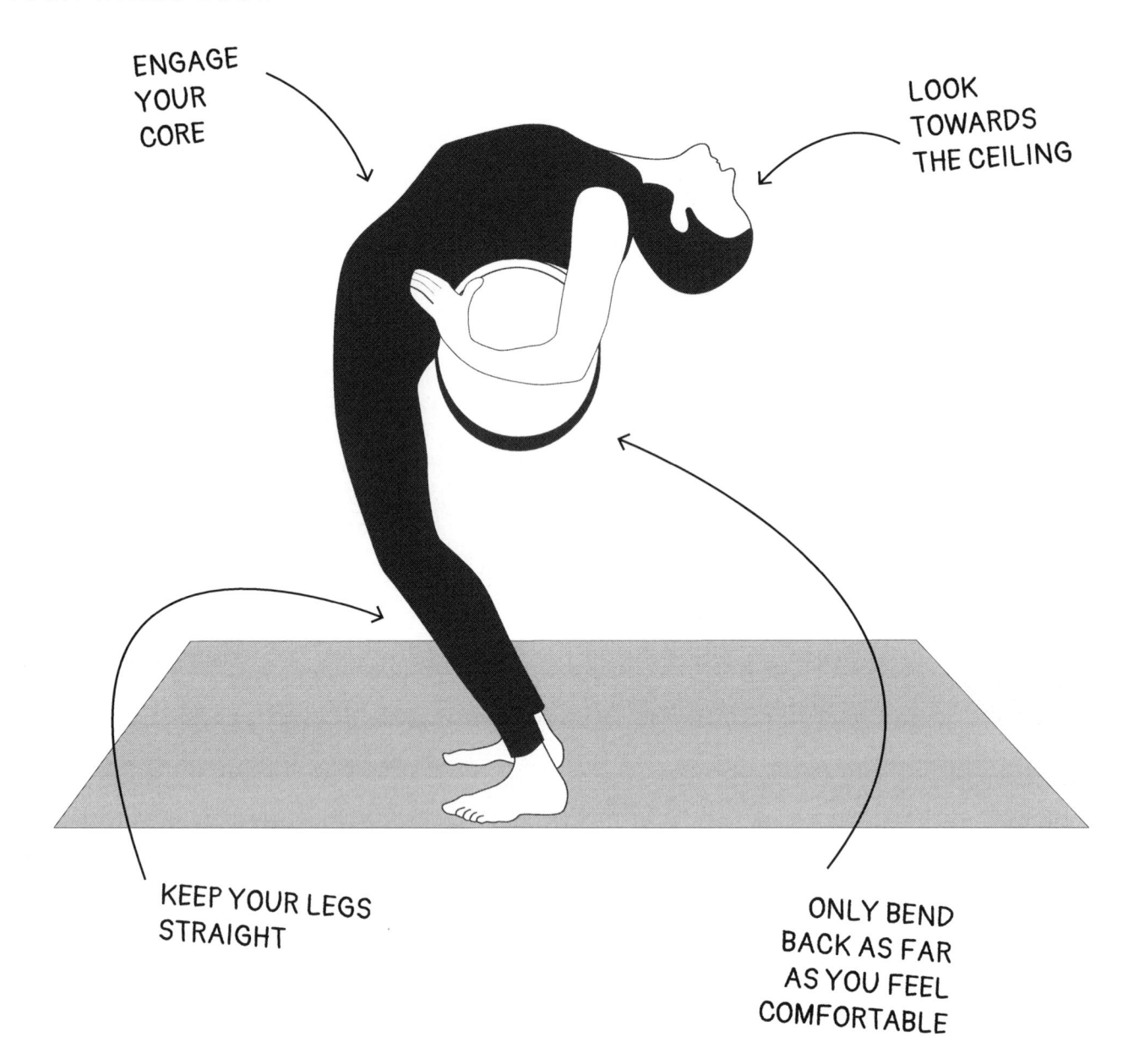

ENGAGE YOUR CORE

LOOK TOWARDS THE CEILING

KEEP YOUR LEGS STRAIGHT

ONLY BEND BACK AS FAR AS YOU FEEL COMFORTABLE

INTERMEDIATE

Standing Backbend

Anuvittasana

The Standing Backbend is a preparatory pose to try before attempting a full backbend. It is perfect for opening up the chest and releasing tension in the neck and shoulders. Using the wheel in this position helps to mobilise the spine and achieve a broader range of movement.

1. Start in a standing position, holding the wheel in the centre of your spine.

2. Keep your core engaged and your legs straight as you slowly bend backwards and wrap your spine over the wheel.

3. Only go as far as you feel comfortable, and then look up to the ceiling as you hold the pose.

TARGETS: SPINE, CORE, HIPS

YOGA WHEEL BOOK

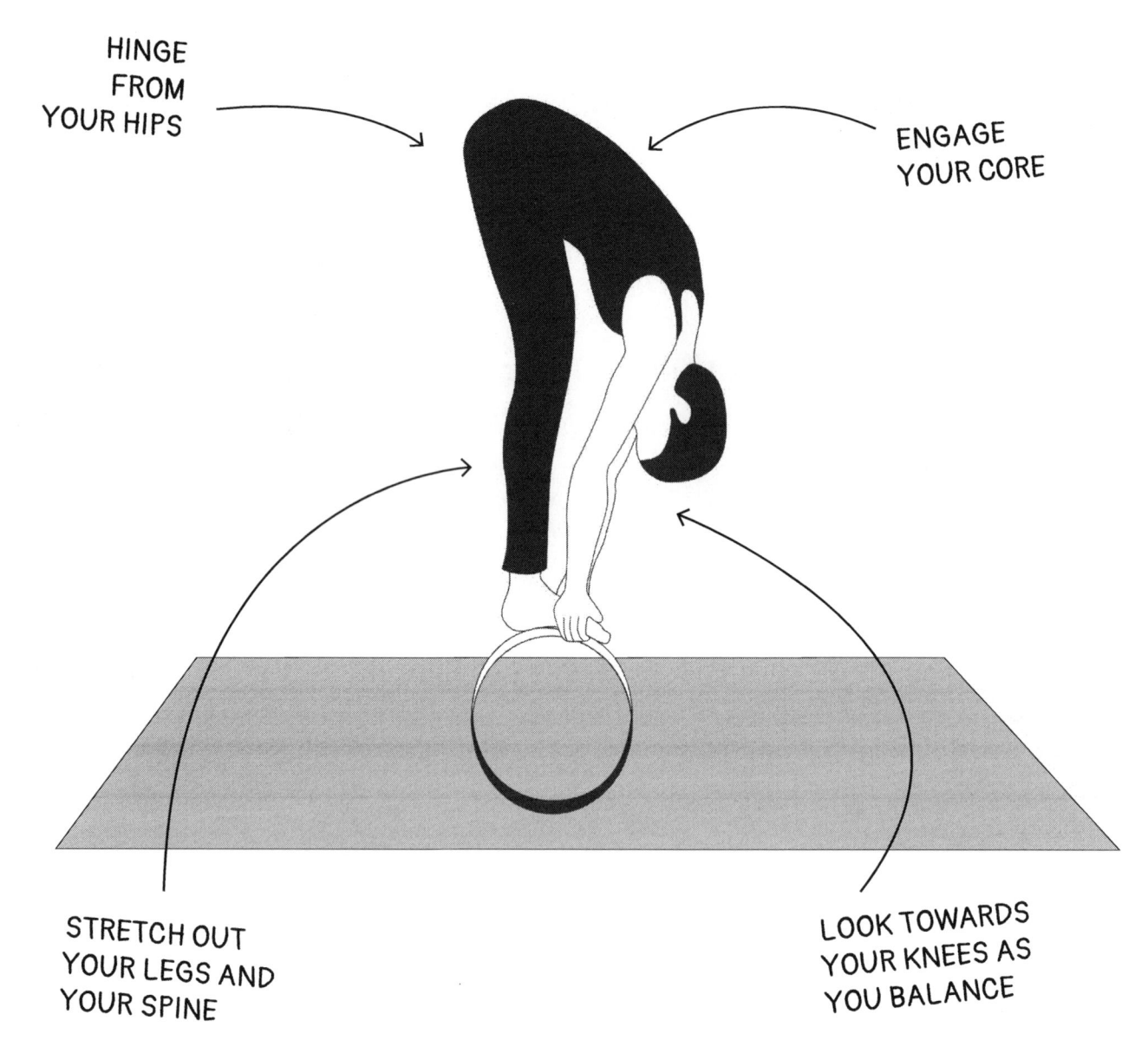

HINGE FROM YOUR HIPS

ENGAGE YOUR CORE

STRETCH OUT YOUR LEGS AND YOUR SPINE

LOOK TOWARDS YOUR KNEES AS YOU BALANCE

INTERMEDIATE

Standing Forward Fold

Padangusthasana

The Standing Forward Fold stretches out the back of the legs and the spine. Standing on the wheel also challenges balance and strength in preparation for more advanced poses.

1. Start in a standing position with your feet hip-width apart and the wheel in front of you.

2. Slowly step both feet onto the wheel, using a wall to help you balance if you need to.

3. Once you feel stable, slowly bend forward, keeping your legs straight and hinging from your hips.

4. Lengthen your arms and grab hold of your toes.

TARGETS: SPINE, CORE, HIPS

YOGA WHEEL BOOK

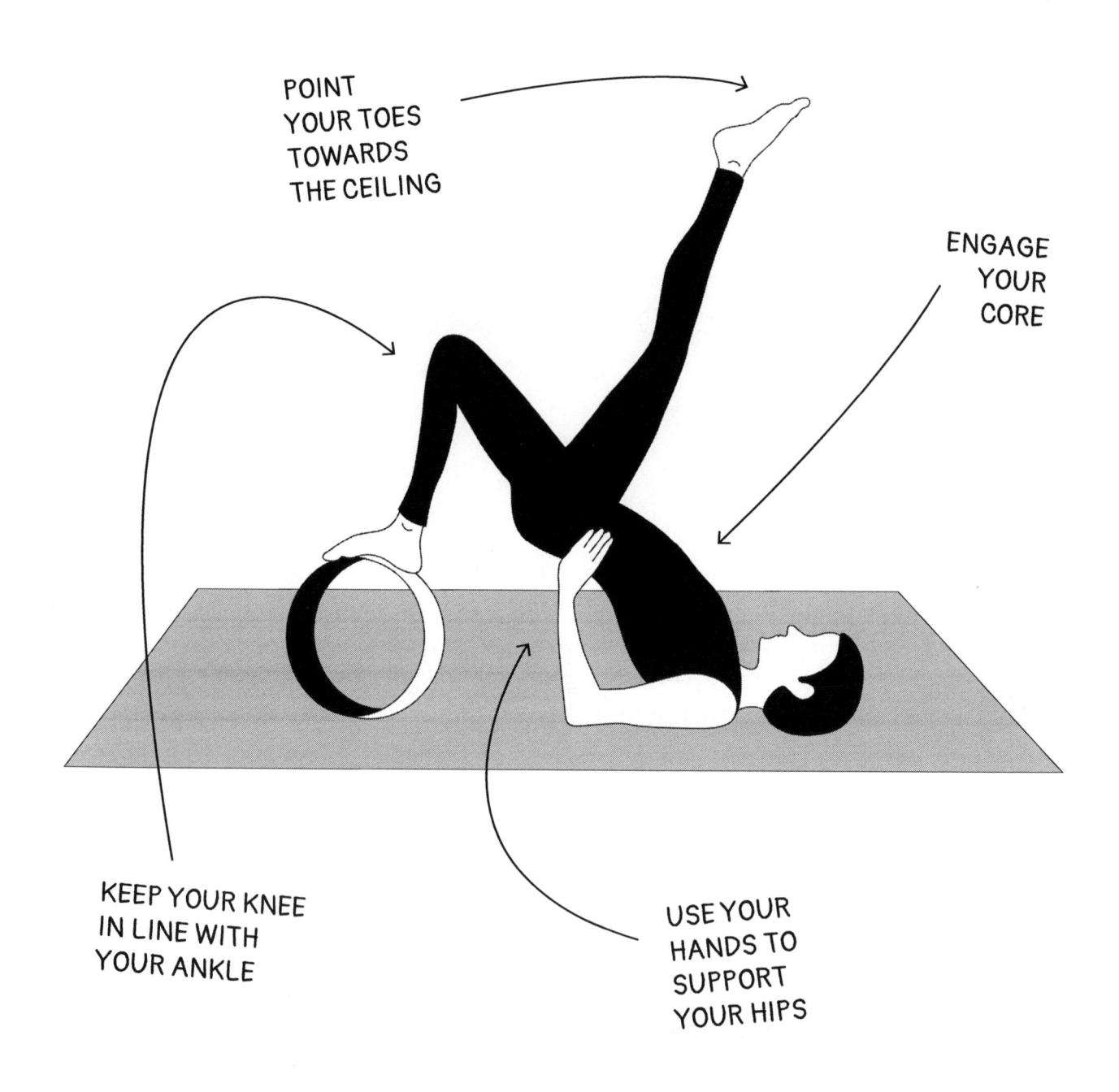

POINT YOUR TOES TOWARDS THE CEILING

ENGAGE YOUR CORE

KEEP YOUR KNEE IN LINE WITH YOUR ANKLE

USE YOUR HANDS TO SUPPORT YOUR HIPS

INTERMEDIATE

One-legged Bridge

Eka Pada Setubandha Sarvangasana

The One-legged Bridge challenges your balance and strength by focusing on one side of the body at a time. Using the wheel in this position requires extra stability.

1. Start by lying on your mat, with your knees bent and the wheel in front of you.

2. Slowly peel your spine off the mat and into a bridge position.

3. Lift both feet onto the wheel and use your hands to support your hips.

4. Lift one leg at a time off the wheel, pointing your toes towards the ceiling.

TARGETS: CORE, CHEST, SHOULDERS, HIP FLEXORS

YOGA WHEEL BOOK

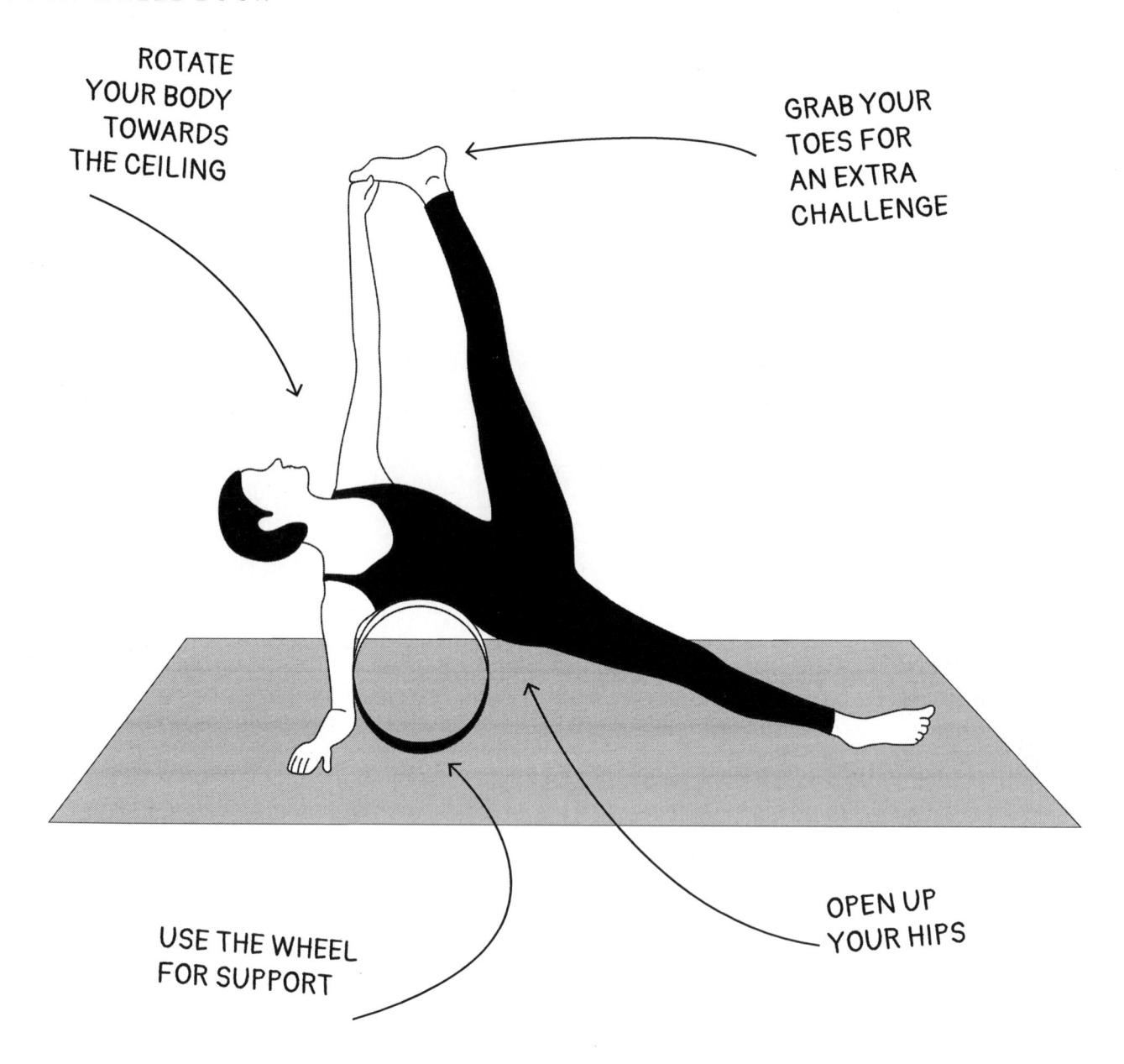

ROTATE YOUR BODY TOWARDS THE CEILING

GRAB YOUR TOES FOR AN EXTRA CHALLENGE

USE THE WHEEL FOR SUPPORT

OPEN UP YOUR HIPS

INTERMEDIATE

One-legged Side Plank

Eka Pada Vasisthasana

The One-legged Side Plank is a great way to target core strength and stability. Using the wheel here gives you additional support to try the more challenging reach towards your toes.

1. Start in a kneeling position with the wheel in the centre of the mat.

2. Bend sideways over the wheel until your forearm rests on the floor and the wheel is underneath your armpit.

3. Extend both of your legs to lift into a full side plank.

4. Rotate your body towards the ceiling, and then lift your left leg off the floor.

5. Reach your left arm towards your leg and grab hold of your toes.

TARGETS: CHEST, SHOULDERS, HIP FLEXORS, CORE

YOGA WHEEL BOOK

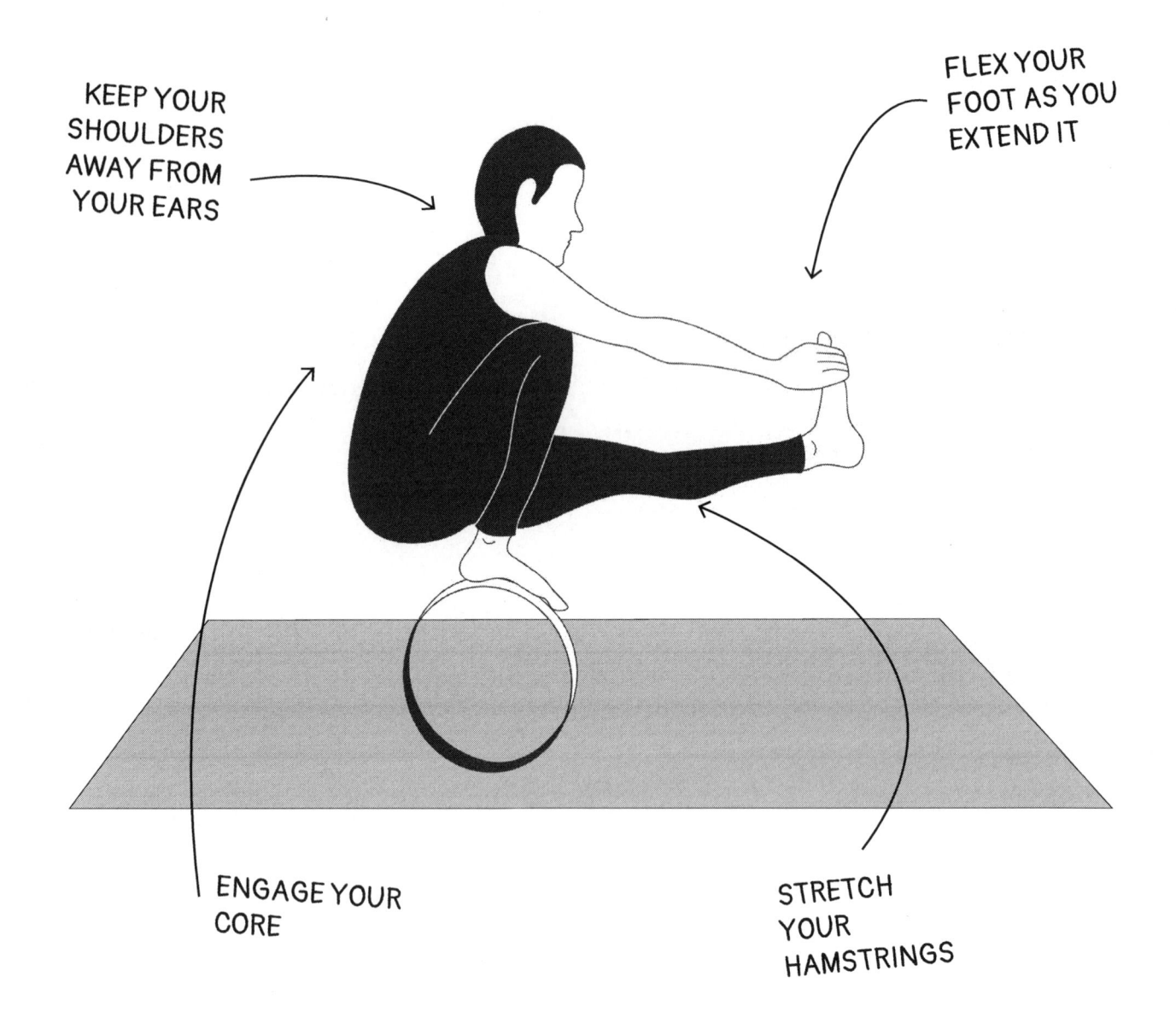

KEEP YOUR SHOULDERS AWAY FROM YOUR EARS

FLEX YOUR FOOT AS YOU EXTEND IT

ENGAGE YOUR CORE

STRETCH YOUR HAMSTRINGS

INTERMEDIATE

Toe Stand

Padangusthasana

The Toe Stand requires a strong core to stay on top of the wheel. It helps to increase flexibility in the hips and improve the posture of the whole body. This position is the perfect way to practice for some of the more advanced balance poses.

1. Start in a seated position with the sole of your right foot on the wheel.

2. Grasp the front of the wheel as you balance, and then bring your left foot onto the wheel. Try to focus on one spot as your feet grasp the wheel.

3. Once you are stable, slowly extend your right foot away from you, flexing your foot.

4. Reach your arms to grab your toes, making sure that your shoulders are away from your ears.

TARGETS: HIPS, BALANCE, POSTURE, HAMSTRINGS

YOGA WHEEL BOOK

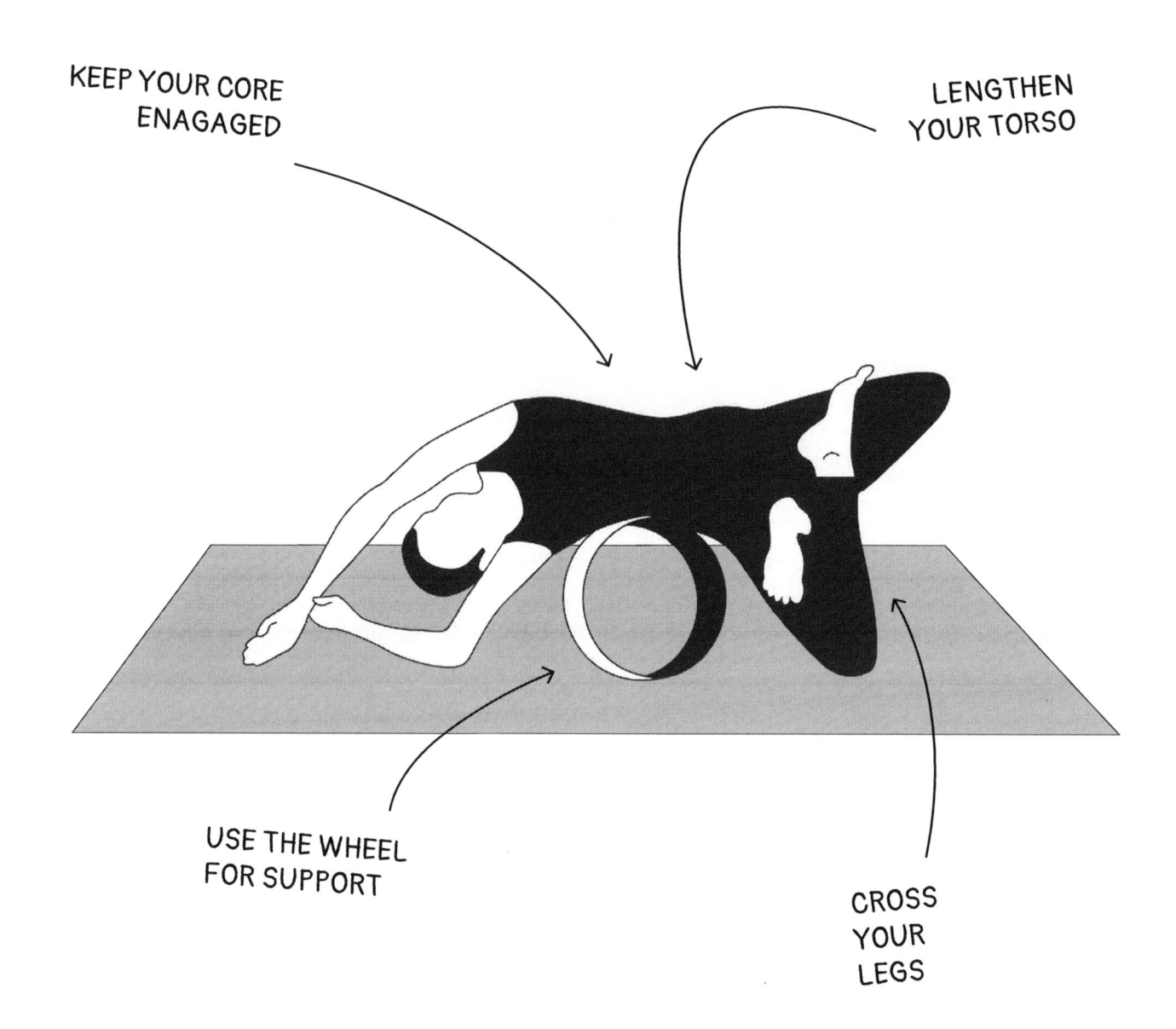

KEEP YOUR CORE ENAGAGED

LENGTHEN YOUR TORSO

USE THE WHEEL FOR SUPPORT

CROSS YOUR LEGS

INTERMEDIATE

Side Bend with Butterfly Legs

Urdhva Hastasana

The Side Bend with Butterfly Legs stretches out the whole body and opens up the ribs. Using the wheel in this position helps to maintain the correct posture and prevents collapsing into the stretch.

1. Start in a kneeling position with the wheel to your right.
2. Reach your arms above your head to lengthen your upper body.
3. Bend over to your right until your side rests on the wheel.
4. Lengthen your arms over the wheel until they reach the mat.
5. Keeping your core engaged and your torso long, fold your legs into a butterfly position.

TARGETS: SIDE, CORE, HIPS, SHOULDERS

YOGA WHEEL BOOK

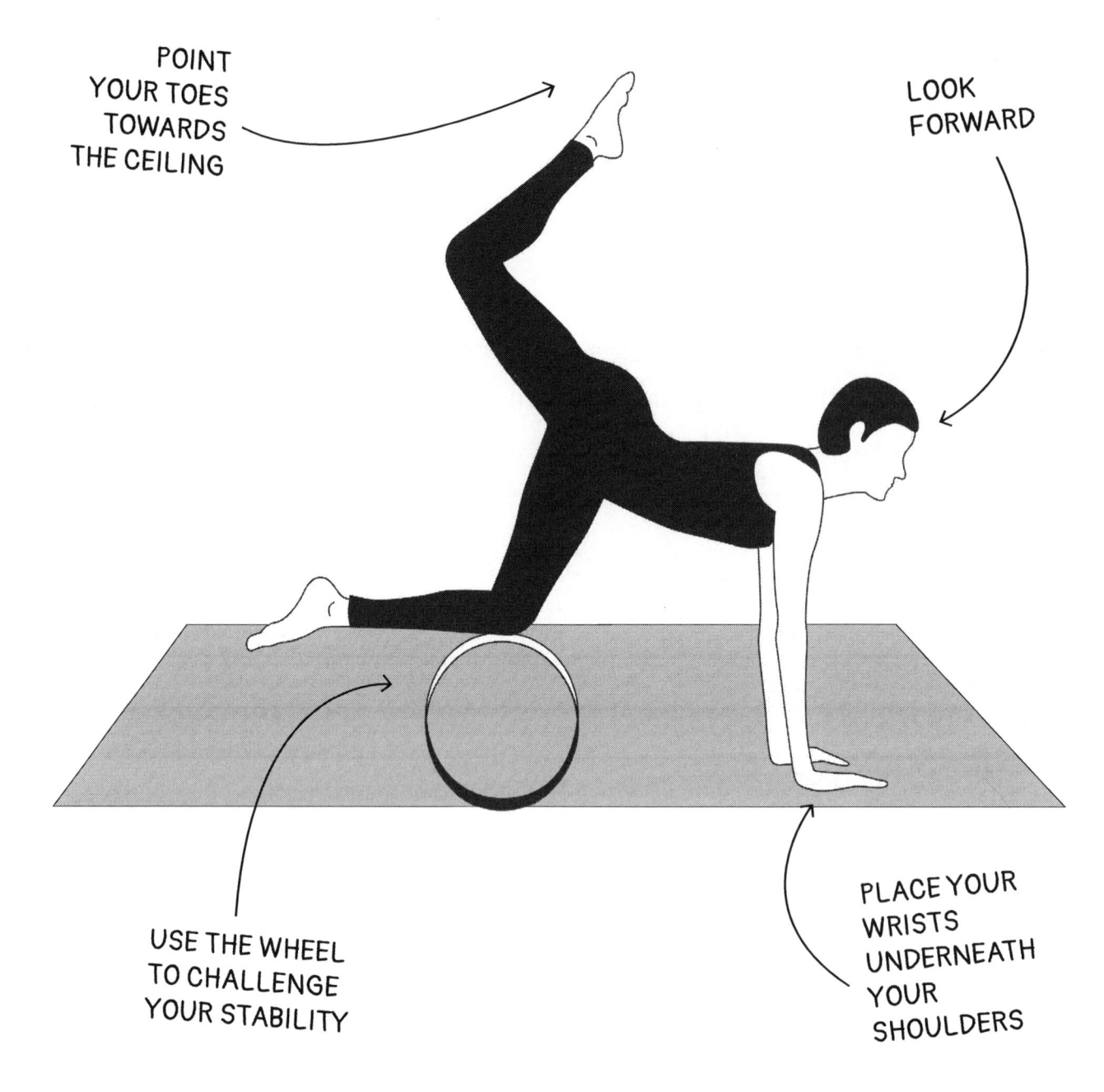

POINT YOUR TOES TOWARDS THE CEILING

LOOK FORWARD

USE THE WHEEL TO CHALLENGE YOUR STABILITY

PLACE YOUR WRISTS UNDERNEATH YOUR SHOULDERS

INTERMEDIATE

Bird Dog

Dandayamana

The Bird Dog improves stability and core strength. It is also a good exercise for relieving lower back pain. Using the wheel in this position makes it more challenging to keep the lower leg stable.

1. Start on all fours in a tabletop position, with the wheel beside your legs.

2. Lift your left knee and place it on the wheel.

3. Lift your right leg up and back, with your toes pointing towards the ceiling.

4. Engage your core and look forward as you hold the pose.

TARGETS: CORE, HIPS, BACK, POSTURE

YOGA WHEEL BOOK

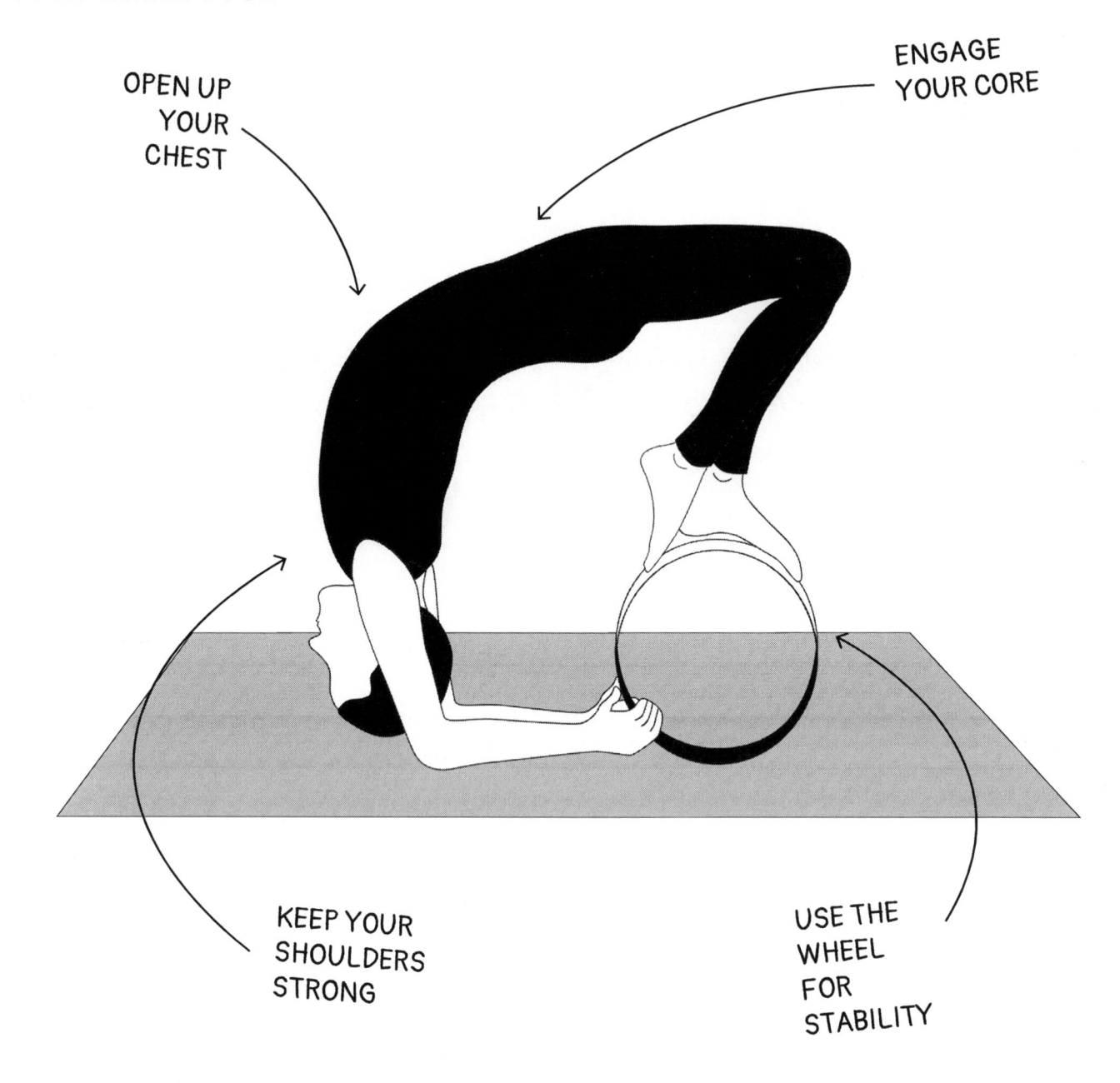

OPEN UP YOUR CHEST

ENGAGE YOUR CORE

KEEP YOUR SHOULDERS STRONG

USE THE WHEEL FOR STABILITY

INTERMEDIATE

Upward Bow

Urdhva Dhanurasana

The Upward Bow requires balance and flexibility. It combines a headstand with a backbend, making it the perfect practice before attempting a full Bow pose. Using the wheel in this position gives you extra stability.

1. Start with your knees and forearms on the floor, holding the wheel with both hands.

2. Come up into a headstand pose and balance on your forearms, holding onto the wheel.

3. Slowly move one leg at a time down onto the wheel.

TARGETS: SPINE, CORE, SHOULDERS

YOGA WHEEL BOOK

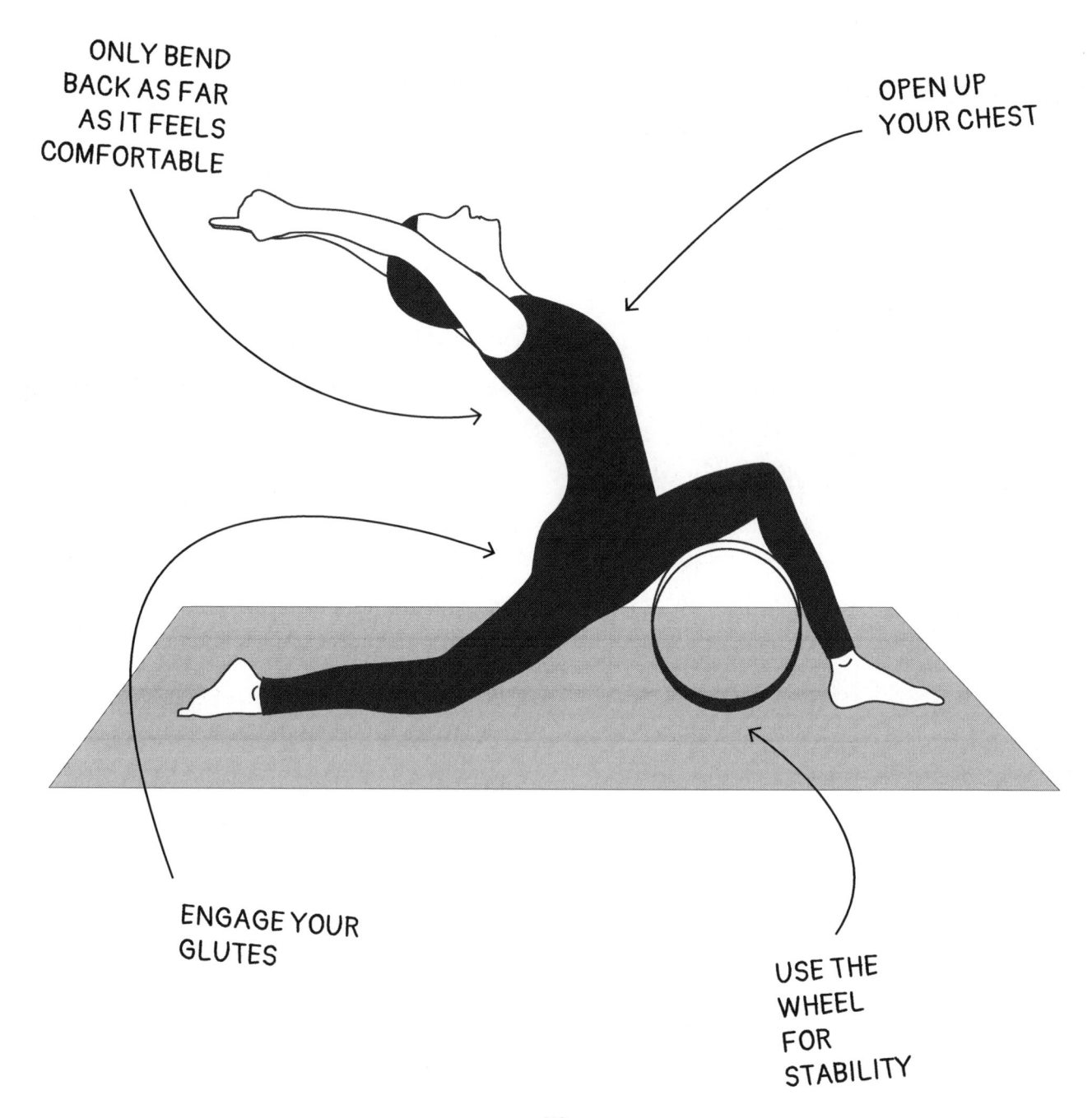

ONLY BEND BACK AS FAR AS IT FEELS COMFORTABLE

OPEN UP YOUR CHEST

ENGAGE YOUR GLUTES

USE THE WHEEL FOR STABILITY

INTERMEDIATE

Seated High Lunge Backbend

Upavistha Ashta Chandrasana Backbend

The Seated High Lunge Backbend is a great way to open up the hips and the chest. It also helps to increase mobility in the spine and work towards more advanced backbends. The wheel provides stability and allows you to get deeper into the stretch.

1. Start in a standing position with the wheel on the mat in front of you.

2. Take a large step forward over the wheel and into a deep lunge.

3. Straighten your back leg and open your chest as you look up to the ceiling.

4. Bring your arms above your head and reach as you bend back into the pose.

TARGETS: HIPS, CHEST, HAMSTRINGS, BACK, GLUTES

YOGA WHEEL BOOK

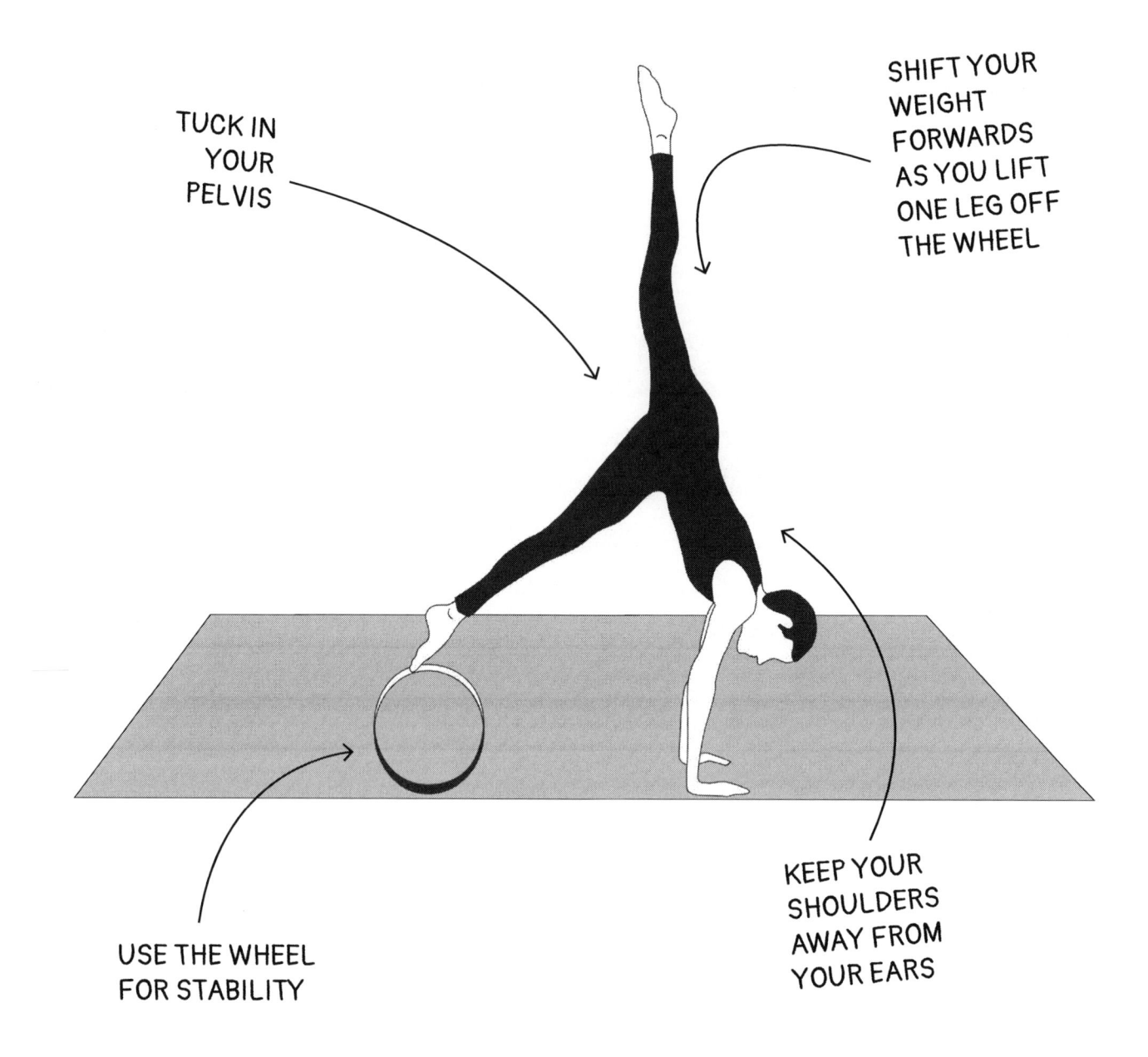

TUCK IN YOUR PELVIS

SHIFT YOUR WEIGHT FORWARDS AS YOU LIFT ONE LEG OFF THE WHEEL

USE THE WHEEL FOR STABILITY

KEEP YOUR SHOULDERS AWAY FROM YOUR EARS

INTERMEDIATE

Pike Handstand

Adho Mukha Vrksasana

The Pike Handstand uses the wheel to help you practice a full handstand. The wheel provides extra stability until you can lift both legs off.

1. Start in a standing position with the wheel behind you on the mat.

2. Bend forwards into a Pike position, and place both hands on the mat in front of you.

3. Slowly lift both of your legs so that they rest on the wheel behind you.

4. Tuck in your pelvis and shift your weight forwards as you lift one leg off the wheel.

TARGETS: CORE, SHOULDERS, CHEST, POSTURE

YOGA WHEEL BOOK

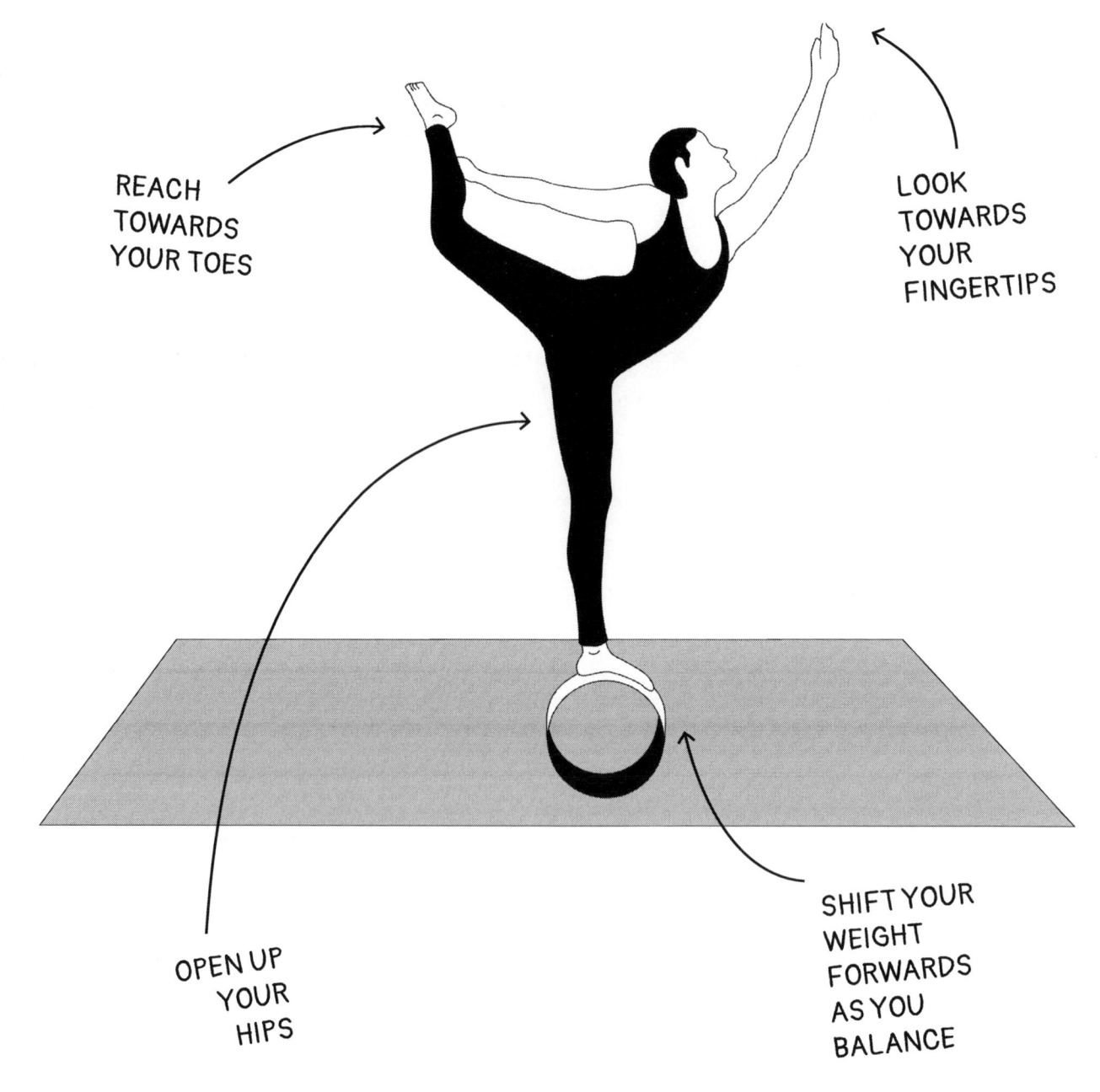

REACH TOWARDS YOUR TOES

LOOK TOWARDS YOUR FINGERTIPS

OPEN UP YOUR HIPS

SHIFT YOUR WEIGHT FORWARDS AS YOU BALANCE

ADVANCED

Dancer Balance

Natarajasana

Once you have mastered the Dancer pose, you can try the Dancer Balance for an extra challenge. Standing on the wheel requires you to stay focused throughout the pose. It's a good idea to practice this pose near a wall in case you lose your balance!

1. Start standing on the mat with the wheel in front of you.

2. Slowly step both feet onto the wheel.

3. Once you are stable on the wheel, gently lift your right leg off, and reach it up and back.

4. Reach behind with your right arm and take hold of your right leg.

5. Stretch your left arm out in front of you and look towards it.

TARGETS: CHEST, SHOULDERS, HIPS, BALANCE

YOGA WHEEL BOOK

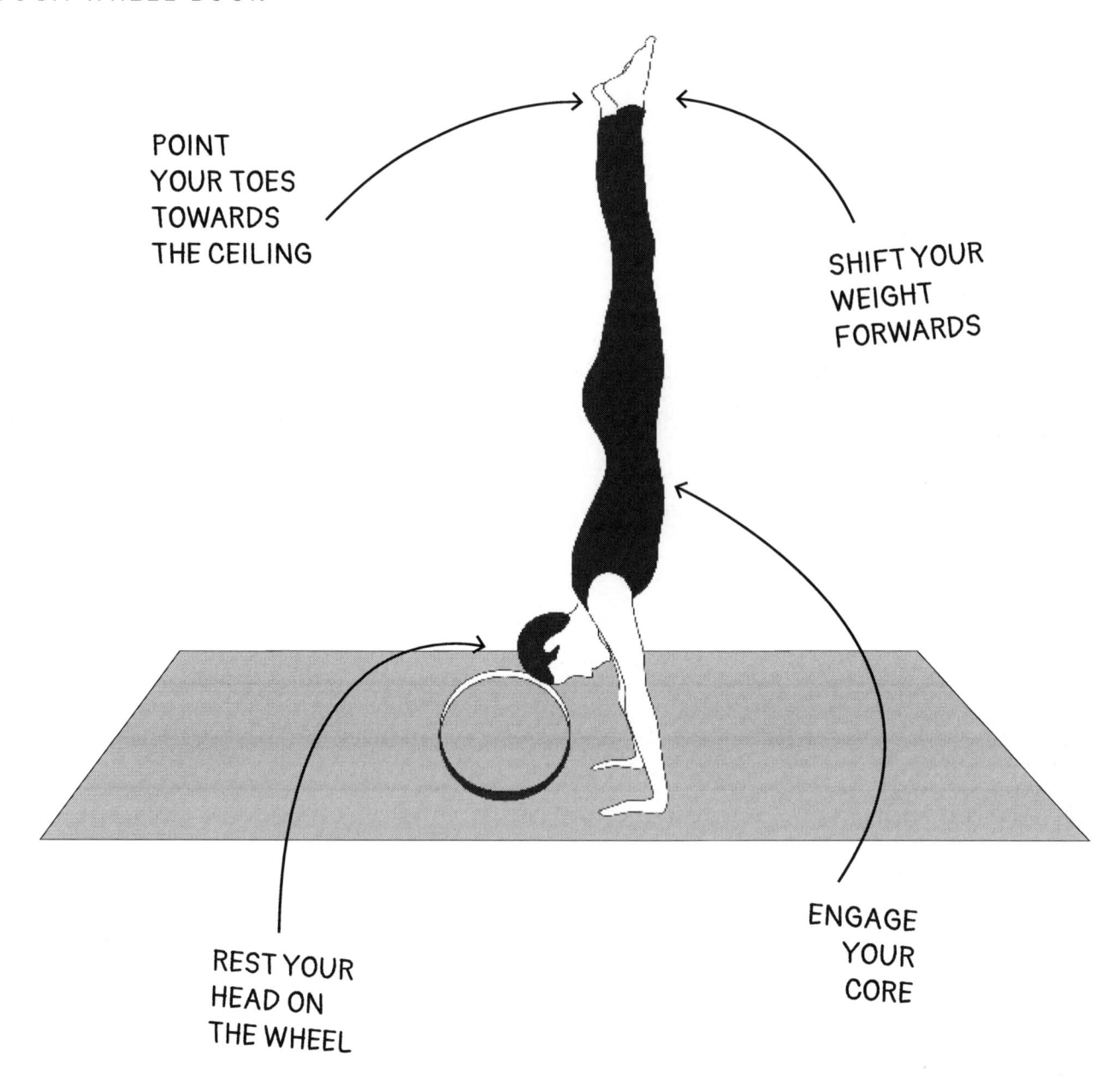

POINT YOUR TOES TOWARDS THE CEILING

SHIFT YOUR WEIGHT FORWARDS

REST YOUR HEAD ON THE WHEEL

ENGAGE YOUR CORE

ADVANCED

Handstand

Adho Mukha Vrksasana

The full Handstand requires strong arms, shoulders and core, as well as mental focus and concentration. Using the wheel to assist you in this pose helps to build confidence and conquer the fear of falling.

1. Start standing on your mat, with the wheel in front of you.

2. Bring your hands to the mat and place them at either side of the wheel.

3. Keeping your legs straight, shift your weight forward to rest your head on the wheel.

4. Come onto the tips of your toes and engage your core, before jumping up into a handstand.

5. Extend your legs up towards the ceiling.

TARGETS: SHOULDERS, CORE, ARMS, BALANCE

YOGA WHEEL BOOK

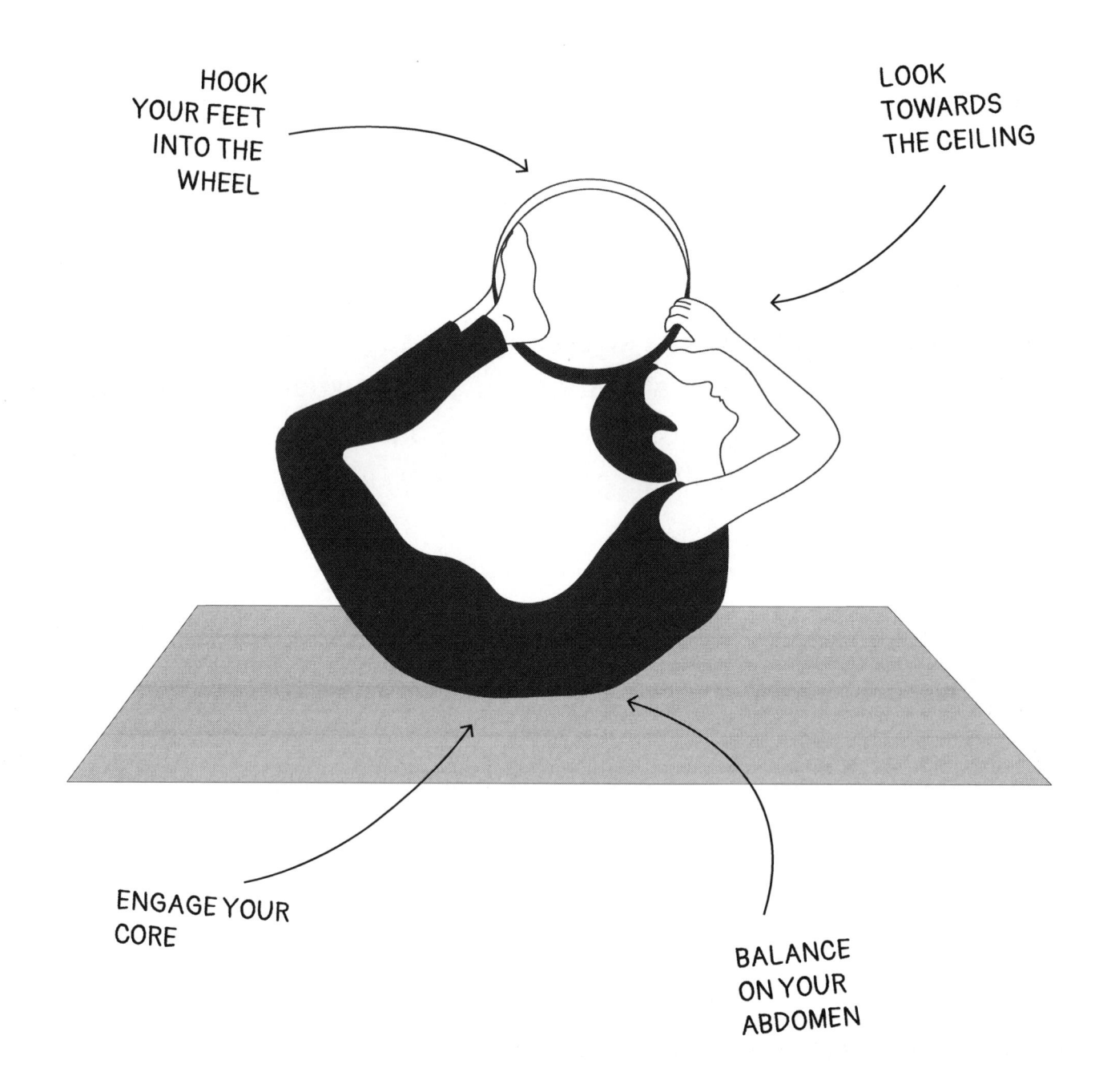

HOOK YOUR FEET INTO THE WHEEL

LOOK TOWARDS THE CEILING

ENGAGE YOUR CORE

BALANCE ON YOUR ABDOMEN

ADVANCED

Bow

Dhanurasana

The Bow is a powerful backbend which balances the entire body on the lower abdomen. It works the core muscles as well as the back. Using the wheel in this position can help you get into a deeper backbend and maintain a good posture.

1. Start lying on your front with your hands in front of you, holding the wheel.

2. Bend your knees and point your toes towards the ceiling as you peel your chest off the mat.

3. Lift your arms above your head and bend backwards until you can hook your feet into the wheel.

4. Engage your core and look up towards the ceiling.

TARGETS: CORE, BACK, FLEXIBILITY, BALANCE

YOGA WHEEL BOOK

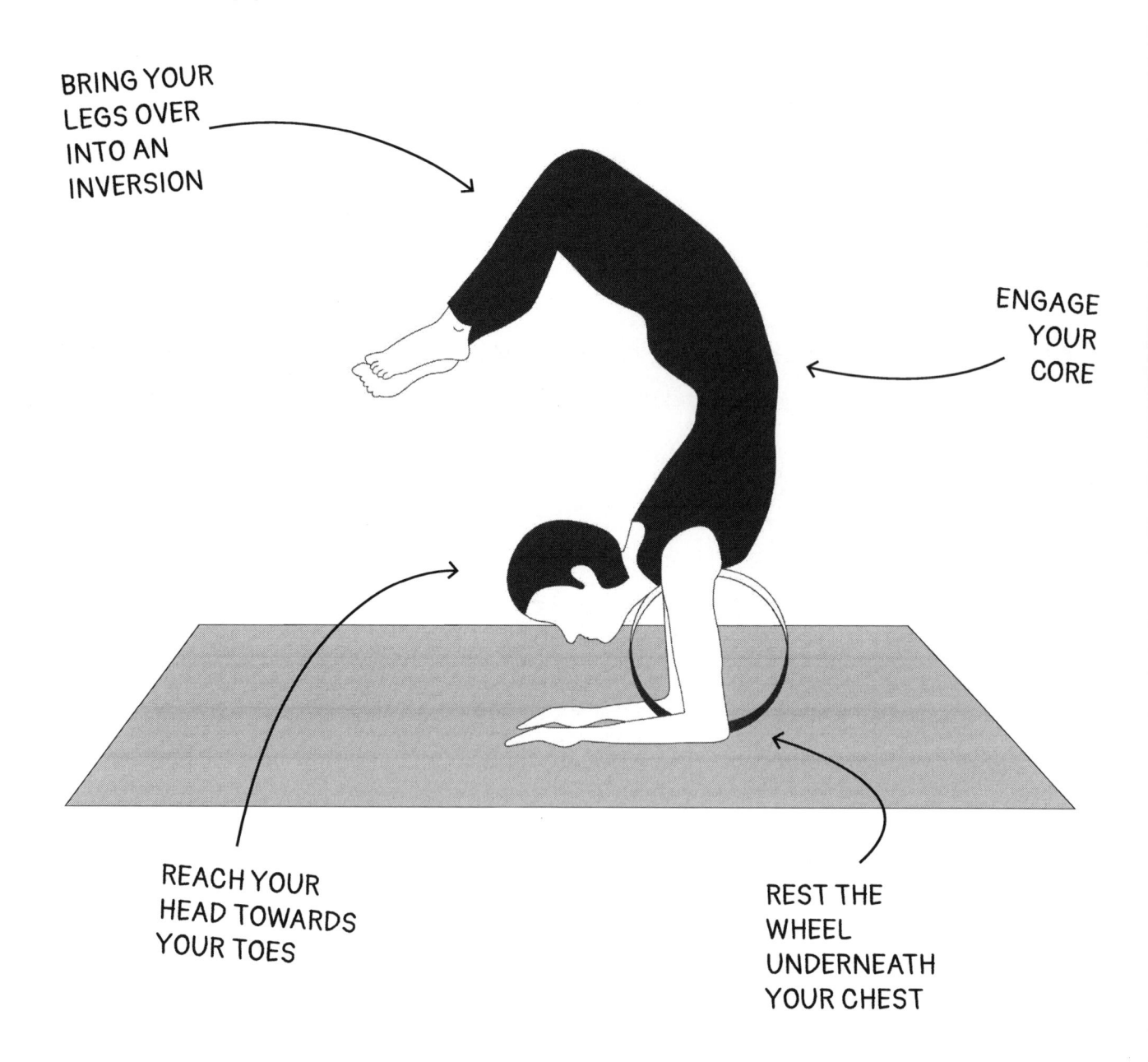

BRING YOUR LEGS OVER INTO AN INVERSION

ENGAGE YOUR CORE

REACH YOUR HEAD TOWARDS YOUR TOES

REST THE WHEEL UNDERNEATH YOUR CHEST

ADVANCED

Scorpion Handstand

Vrschikasana

The Scorpion Handstand requires good core strength and shoulder mobility. Using the wheel can offer extra support as your work towards achieving the full pose.

1. Start by kneeling on the mat with the wheel in front of you.

2. Place your elbows either side of the wheel and lift into a handstand, resting the wheel underneath your chest.

3. Bring your legs over into an inversion.

4. Lift your head off the mat and reach it towards your toes.

TARGETS: CORE, FLEXIBILITY, SPINE, SHOULDERS

YOGA WHEEL BOOK

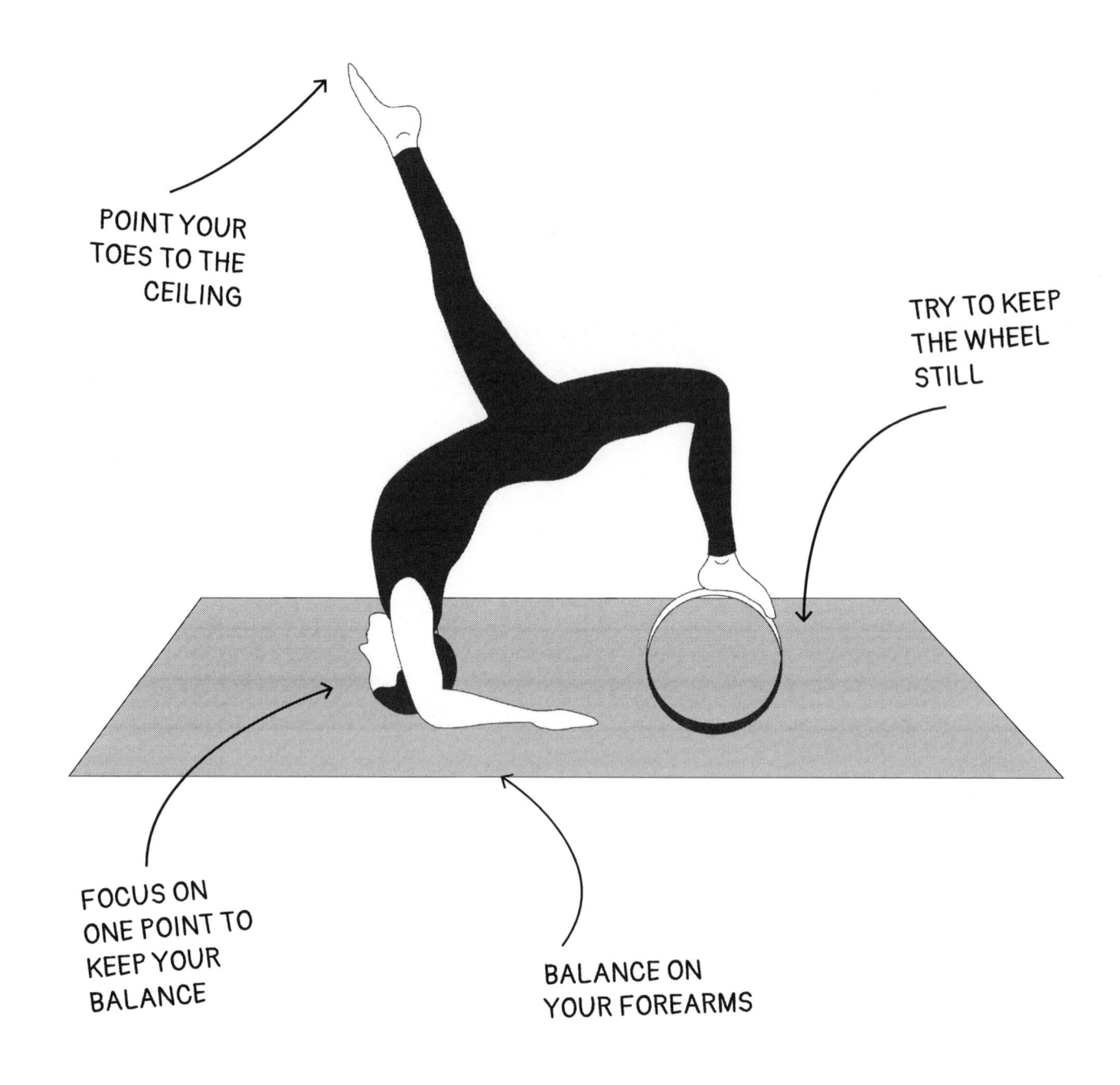

POINT YOUR TOES TO THE CEILING

TRY TO KEEP THE WHEEL STILL

FOCUS ON ONE POINT TO KEEP YOUR BALANCE

BALANCE ON YOUR FOREARMS

ADVANCED

One-legged Upward Bow

Eka Pada Urdhva Dhanurasana

The One-legged Upward Bow challenges your balance and strength. Lifting one leg off the wheel requires focus to keep the wheel from moving.

1. Start with your knees and forearms on the floor, holding the wheel with both hands.

2. Come up into a headstand pose and balance on your forearms, holding onto the wheel.

3. Slowly move one leg at a time down onto the wheel.

4. Once you are stable, slowly lift one leg off the wheel and point your toes to the ceiling.

TARGETS: SHOULDERS, LOWER BACK, CORE

YOGA WHEEL BOOK

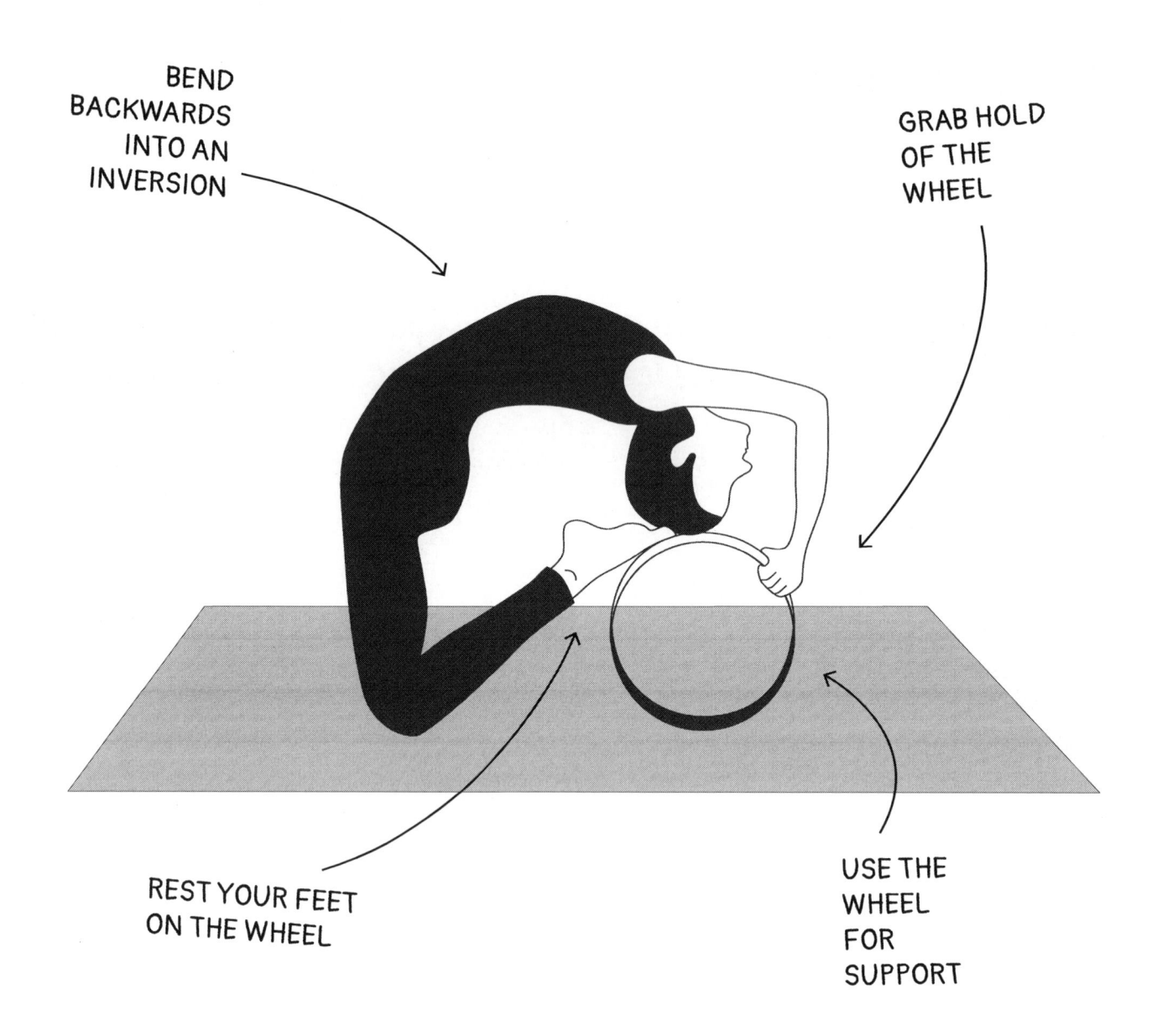

BEND BACKWARDS INTO AN INVERSION

GRAB HOLD OF THE WHEEL

REST YOUR FEET ON THE WHEEL

USE THE WHEEL FOR SUPPORT

ADVANCED

Floating Camel

Ustrasana

The Floating Camel is an advanced variation of the Camel pose, where your body balances on the edge of your feet. The deep backbend also challenges the quads and core. Using the wheel in this position can assist with balance and help you to get into the pose correctly.

1. Start in a kneeling position on your mat, with the wheel directly behind you.

2. Raise your legs so that your feet are resting on the wheel.

3. Bend backwards into an inversion until your head is also resting on the wheel next to your toes.

4. Bring your arms behind your head and grab hold of the wheel.

TARGETS: FLEXIBILITY, SPINE, CORE, CHEST, KNEES

YOGA WHEEL BOOK

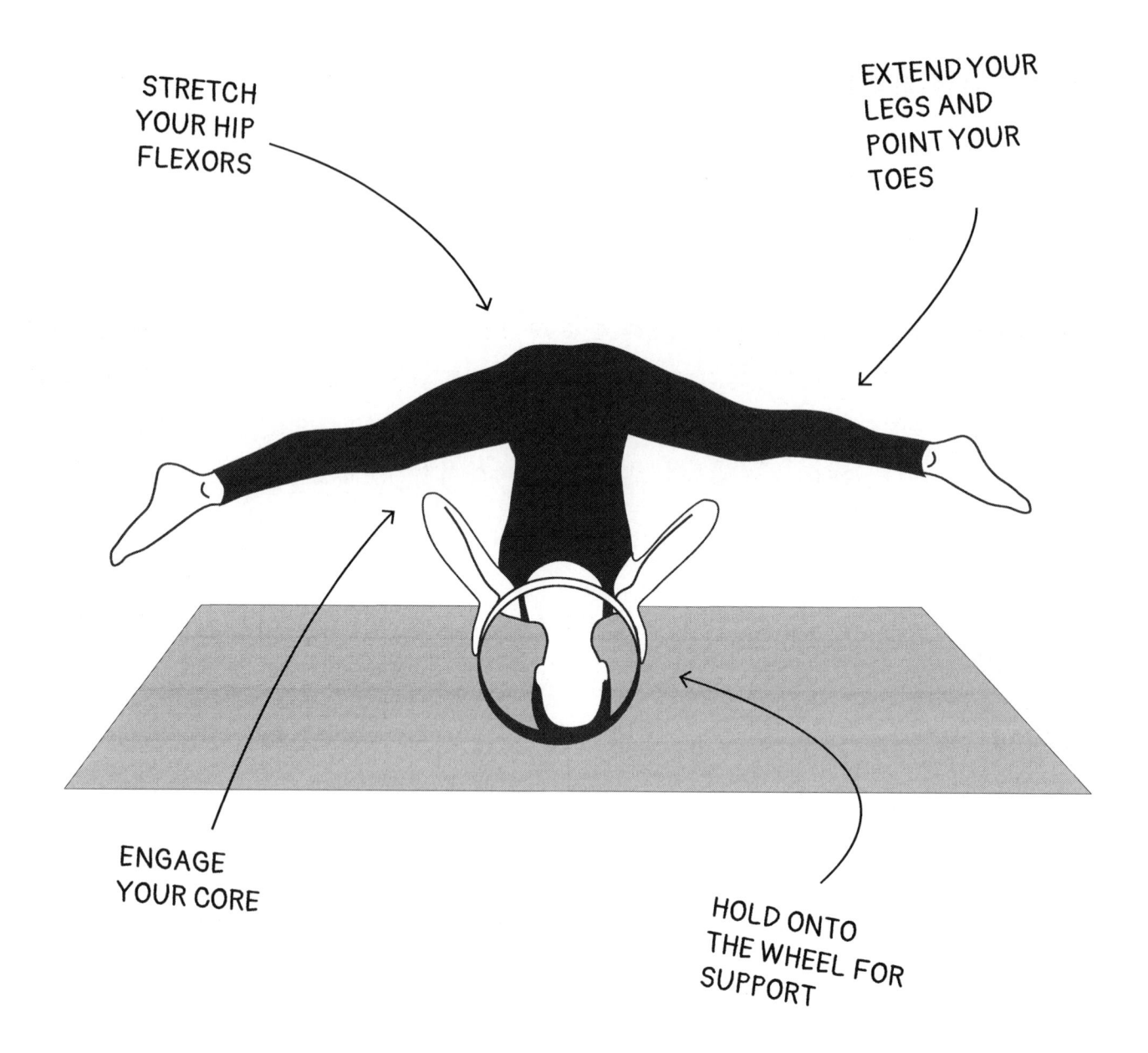

STRETCH YOUR HIP FLEXORS

EXTEND YOUR LEGS AND POINT YOUR TOES

ENGAGE YOUR CORE

HOLD ONTO THE WHEEL FOR SUPPORT

ADVANCED

Headstand with Wide Legs

Salamba Sirsasana Konasana

Once you feel confident and stable in a full headstand, the Headstand with Wide Legs variation is a great way to challenge yourself. The wheel acts as a support and also allows you to practice lifting your hands off the floor.

1. Start by kneeling on your mat, with your hands on the wheel in front of you.

2. Bend forwards so that your head is resting on the mat.

3. Extend your legs up into a full headstand, with your toes pointing towards the ceiling.

4. Once you are confident in the headstand, engage your core and slowly spread your legs out to the side.

TARGETS: ARMS, SHOULDERS, CORE, THIGHS, HIP FLEXORS

YOGA WHEEL BOOK

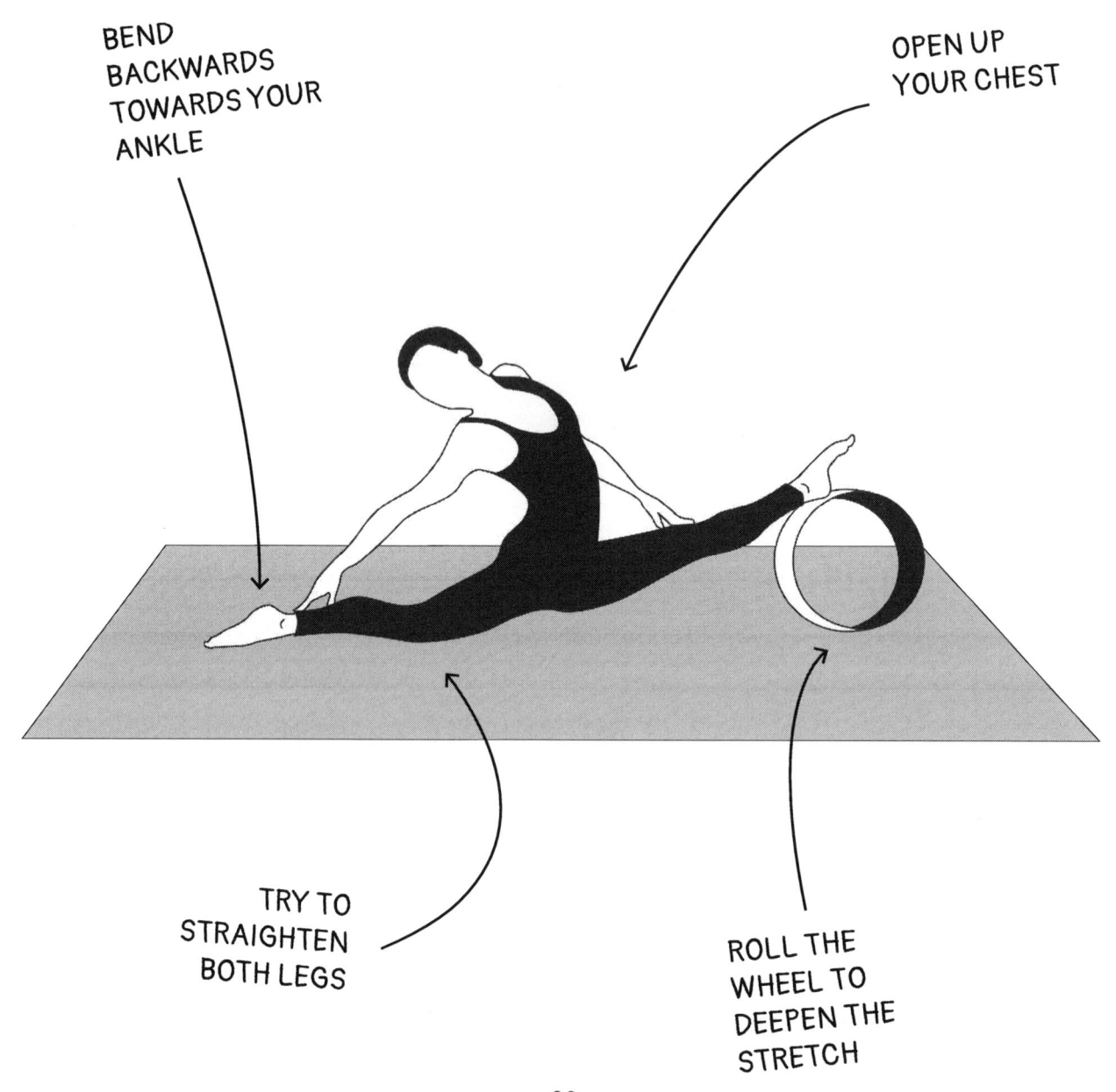

BEND BACKWARDS TOWARDS YOUR ANKLE

OPEN UP YOUR CHEST

TRY TO STRAIGHTEN BOTH LEGS

ROLL THE WHEEL TO DEEPEN THE STRETCH

ADVANCED

Splits

Hanumanasana

The Splits requires strength, flexibility and balance. Using the wheel to help you practice this pose can make it more accessible. You can roll the wheel backwards and forwards in this position to deepen the stretch.

1. Start on the mat, with your right leg forward and your toes pointing up.

2. Keep your right knee slightly bent and your hands on the mat, as you bring your left knee to the mat.

3. Gently move the wheel under your right ankle and try to straighten both legs.

4. For a deeper stretch, bend backwards and reach your right arm towards your left ankle.

TARGETS: HAMSTRINGS, QUADS, PELVIS, HIPS, BACK, CORE, FLEXIBILITY

YOGA WHEEL BOOK

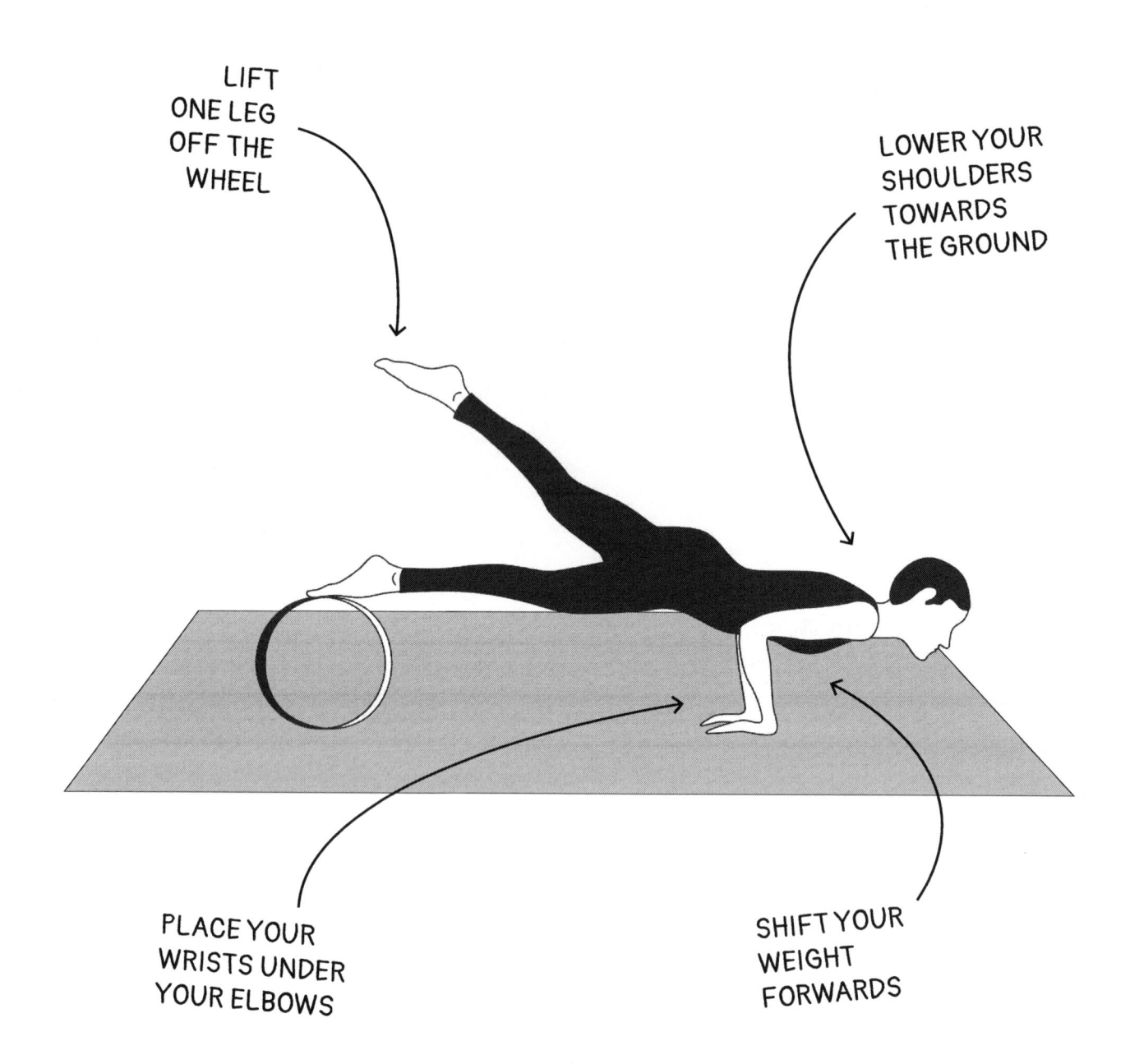

LIFT ONE LEG OFF THE WHEEL

LOWER YOUR SHOULDERS TOWARDS THE GROUND

PLACE YOUR WRISTS UNDER YOUR ELBOWS

SHIFT YOUR WEIGHT FORWARDS

ADVANCED

One-legged Peacock

Eka Pada Mayurasana

The One-legged Peacock is an intense arm balance that helps develop your core strength. Using the wheel in this variation allows you to work towards lifting both legs into a full Peacock pose.

1. Start in a High Plank position with the wheel underneath your shins.

2. Walk your hands towards your chest, so that your wrists are underneath your elbows.

3. Bend your elbows and shift your weight forwards. Then lower towards the ground as you lift one leg off of the wheel.

TARGETS: ARMS, SHOULDERS, CORE, BALANCE

YOGA WHEEL BOOK

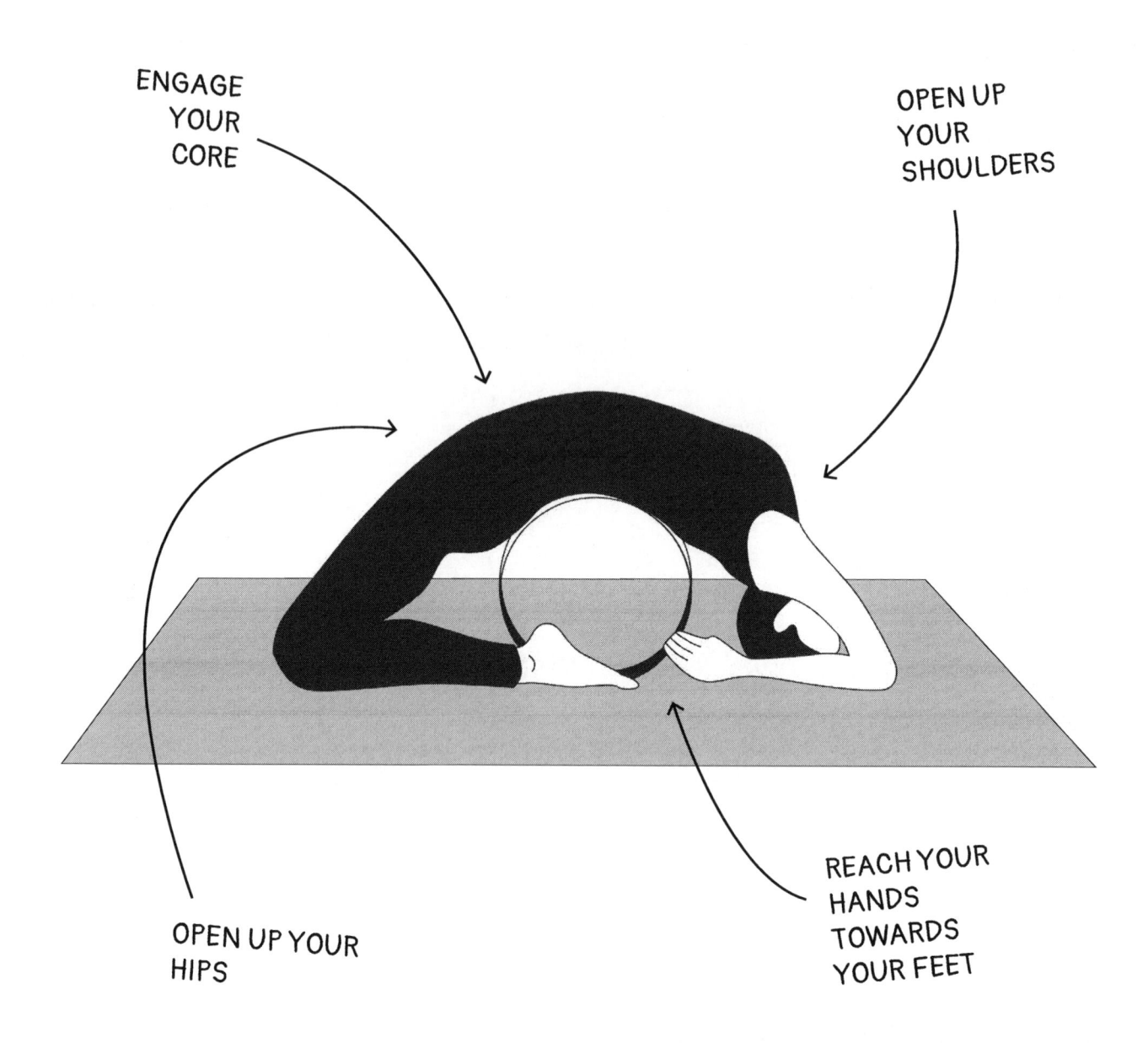

ENGAGE YOUR CORE

OPEN UP YOUR SHOULDERS

OPEN UP YOUR HIPS

REACH YOUR HANDS TOWARDS YOUR FEET

ADVANCED

Pigeon

Kapotasana

The Pigeon is an advanced backbend that requires core strength, strong hip flexors and open shoulders.

1. Start in a kneeling position with the wheel in the centre of your spine.

2. Lift your hips and bend backwards over the wheel, opening up your chest.

3. Reach your arms back behind your head and grab hold of the wheel.

4. Rest your head on the floor and reach your hands towards your feet.

TARGETS: CORE, HIPS, SHOULDERS, BACK, CHEST, FLEXIBILITY

YOGA WHEEL BOOK

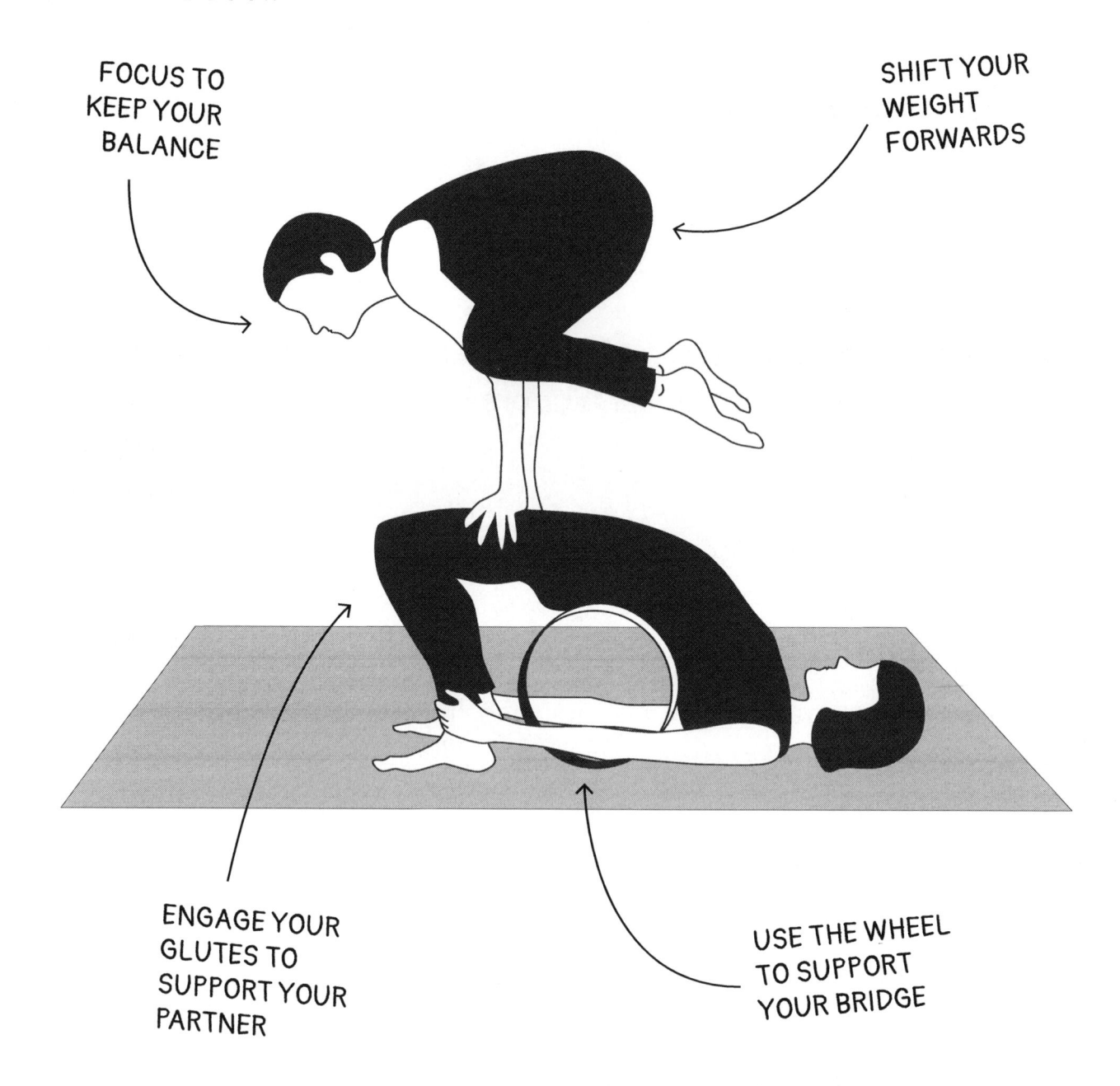

FOCUS TO KEEP YOUR BALANCE

SHIFT YOUR WEIGHT FORWARDS

ENGAGE YOUR GLUTES TO SUPPORT YOUR PARTNER

USE THE WHEEL TO SUPPORT YOUR BRIDGE

Bridge and Crow

Setu Bandha Sarvangasana and Bakasana

The Bridge and Crow is partner variation of an arm balance that requires good core strength. Practising with a partner can challenge your balance and focus. The wheel encourages your partner to reach a higher bridge pose and offers extra stability as they hold your weight.

1. Allow your partner to come into a bridge position with hands reaching forwards to their ankles, and the wheel supporting their back.

2. Stand onto your partner's thighs and move into a squat position, with your feet together and your knees wide apart.

3. Bend forward to grip your shoulders with your knees, and then place your palms on your partner's thighs.

4. Shift your weight forward off your toes and balance on your arms.

TARGETS: CORE, BACK, ARMS, BALANCE

YOGA WHEEL BOOK

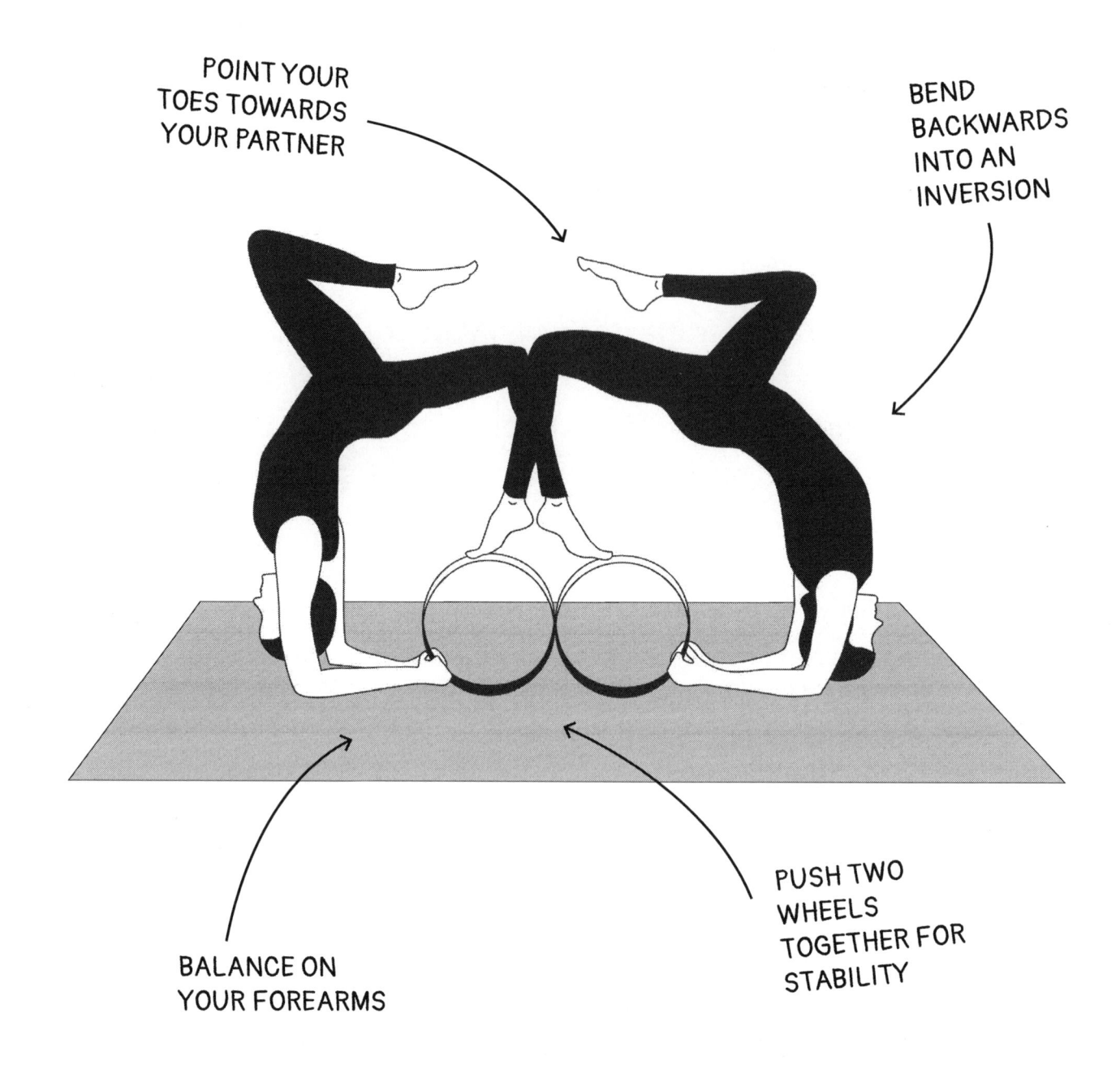

POINT YOUR TOES TOWARDS YOUR PARTNER

BEND BACKWARDS INTO AN INVERSION

BALANCE ON YOUR FOREARMS

PUSH TWO WHEELS TOGETHER FOR STABILITY

Half Feathered Peacock

Ardha Pincha Mayurasana Padanguli

The Half Feathered Peacock allows you to practice balance and stability with a partner before attempting the full pose. Using two wheels pushed together creates a sturdy base. Practising this pose with a partner can help you work towards achieving it without support.

1. Start on all fours opposite your partner, with your forearms resting on the ground. Then take hold of the wheel in front of you.

2. Lift your legs towards the ceiling to balance on your forearms. It helps to look down at the mat to keep your balance.

3. Bend over into an inversion and bring one foot down onto the wheel.

4. Bend your other leg and point your toes towards your partner.

TARGETS: CHEST, CORE, ARMS, SHOULDERS, HIPS

YOGA WHEEL BOOK

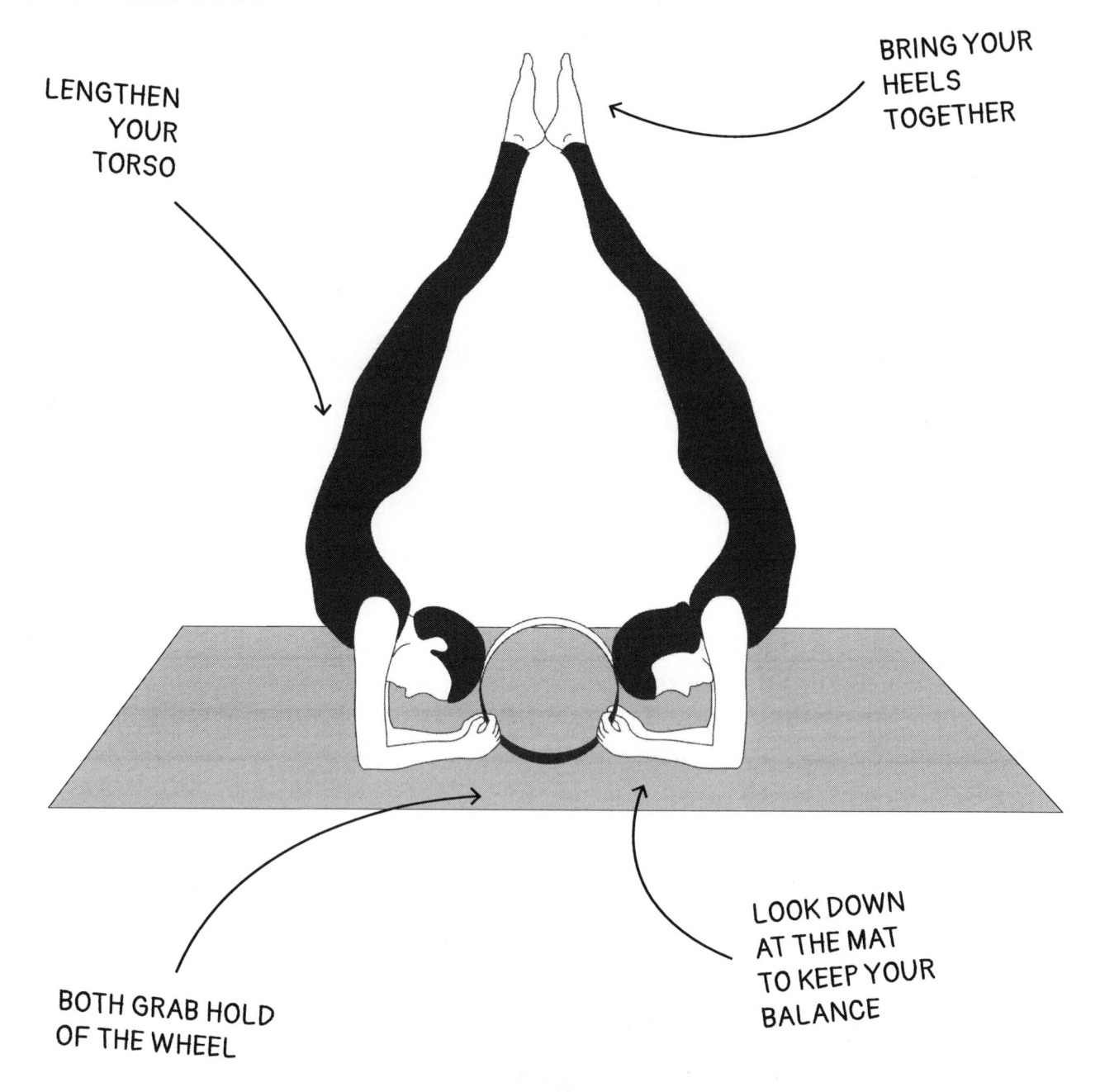

LENGTHEN YOUR TORSO

BRING YOUR HEELS TOGETHER

BOTH GRAB HOLD OF THE WHEEL

LOOK DOWN AT THE MAT TO KEEP YOUR BALANCE

Double Feathered Peacock

Pincha Mayurasana

The Double Feathered Peacock is a forearm inversion that requires core strength and balance. Practising with a partner can give you both stability and help you overcome the fear of falling. The wheel acts as an anchor for you both and assists in achieving perfect form. It works best if you are a similar height and weight to your partner.

1. Start opposite your partner on all fours, with your forearms resting on the ground. Then both grab hold of the wheel in front of you.

2. Lift your legs towards the ceiling to balance on your forearms. It helps to look down at the mat to keep your balance.

3. Bring your heels together and lengthen your torso as you both balance.

4. Make sure that you both come out of the pose at the same time.

TARGETS: CHEST, CORE, ARMS, SHOULDERS, HIPS

YOGA WHEEL BOOK

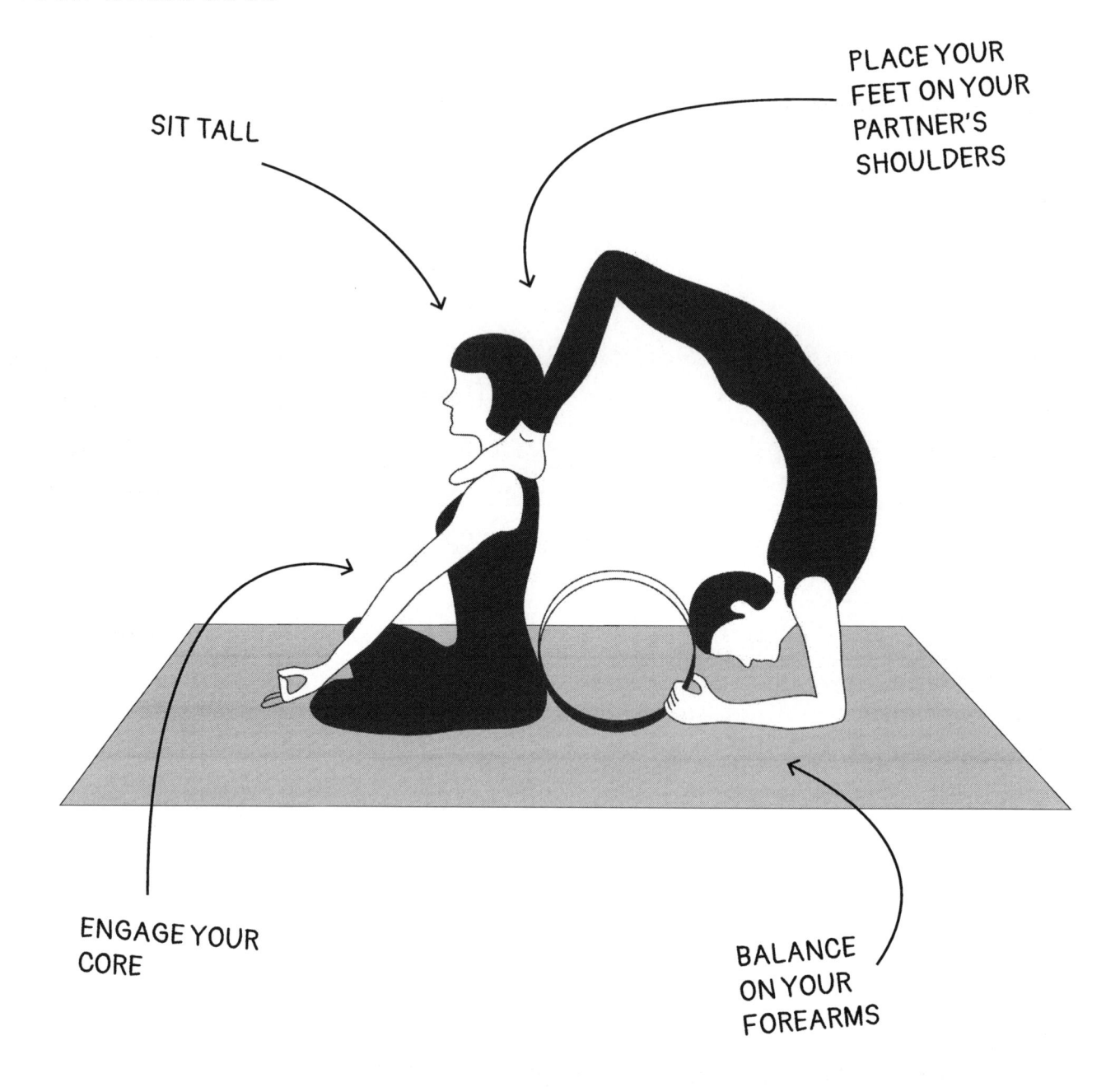

SIT TALL

PLACE YOUR
FEET ON YOUR
PARTNER'S
SHOULDERS

ENGAGE YOUR
CORE

BALANCE
ON YOUR
FOREARMS

PARTNER

Scorpion Handstand Prep

Vrschikasana Prep Uttanasana

The Scorpion Handstand Prep with a partner can give you extra stability as you work towards a full backbend. The wheel offers support for your head, as you rest your feet on your partner's shoulders to perfect the pose. Your partner can also practice core strength and good posture in this pose.

1. Start by kneeling on the mat, with your partner facing away from you.

2. Place the wheel in between you both.

3. Place your elbows either side of the wheel and lift into a handstand position. Then bring your head to rest on the side of the wheel.

4. Bring your legs over into an inversion and place your feet on your partner's shoulders.

TARGETS: CORE, FLEXIBILITY, SPINE, SHOULDERS, POSTURE

YOGA WHEEL BOOK

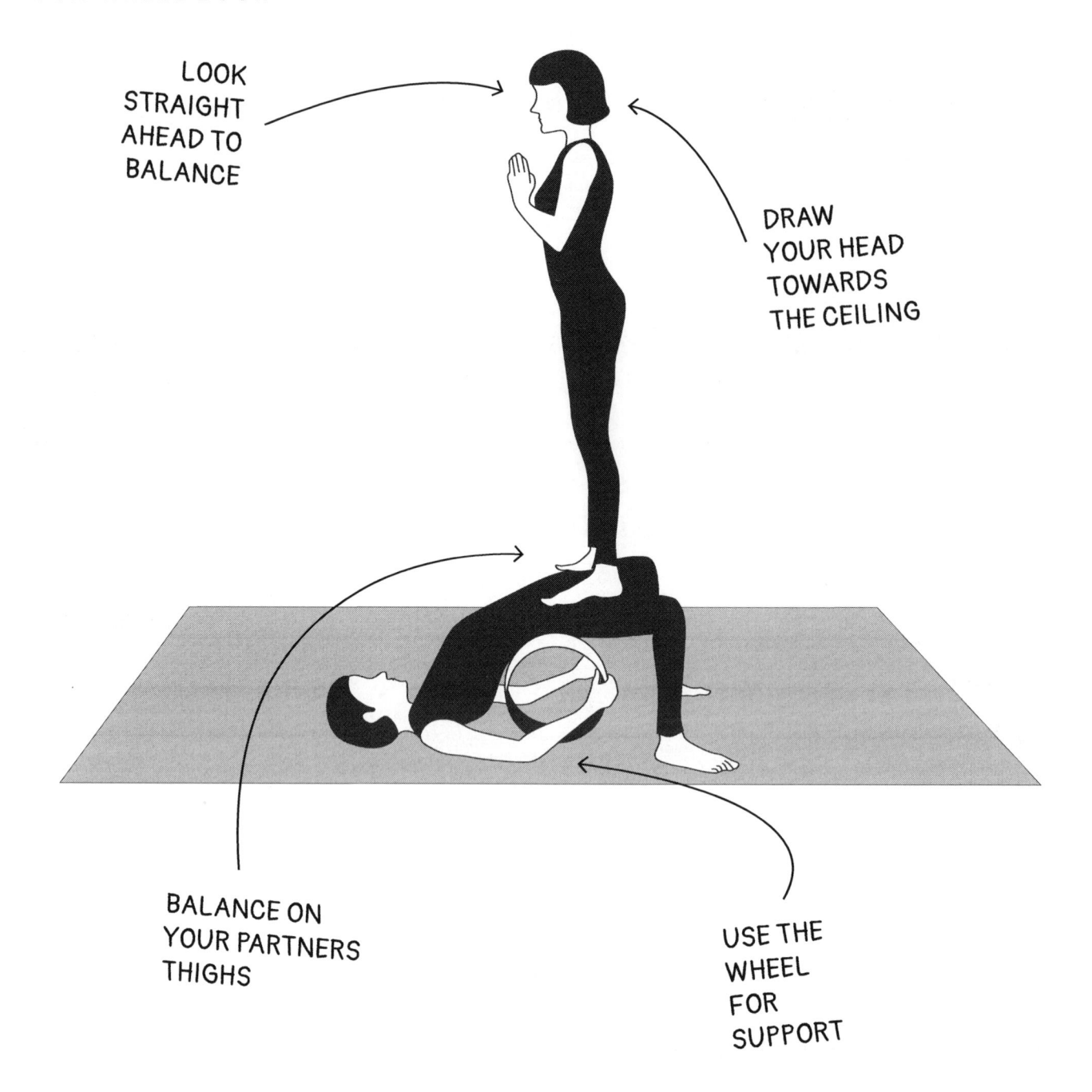

LOOK STRAIGHT AHEAD TO BALANCE

DRAW YOUR HEAD TOWARDS THE CEILING

BALANCE ON YOUR PARTNERS THIGHS

USE THE WHEEL FOR SUPPORT

Bridge and Standing Balance

Setu Bandha Sarvangasana and Pranamasana

The Bridge and Standing Balance requires both partners to practice mental focus and awareness. The wheel offers stability to the partner in a bridge position, while the partner standing on top can practice good posture and balance.

1. Allow your partner to get into a bridge position, with the wheel underneath their back.

2. Standing facing your partner, slowly step on to their thighs, with your toes resting just below their pelvis.

3. Find your balance, draw your head towards the ceiling and bring your hands into prayer as you balance.

TARGETS: BALANCE, BACK, CORE, HIPS

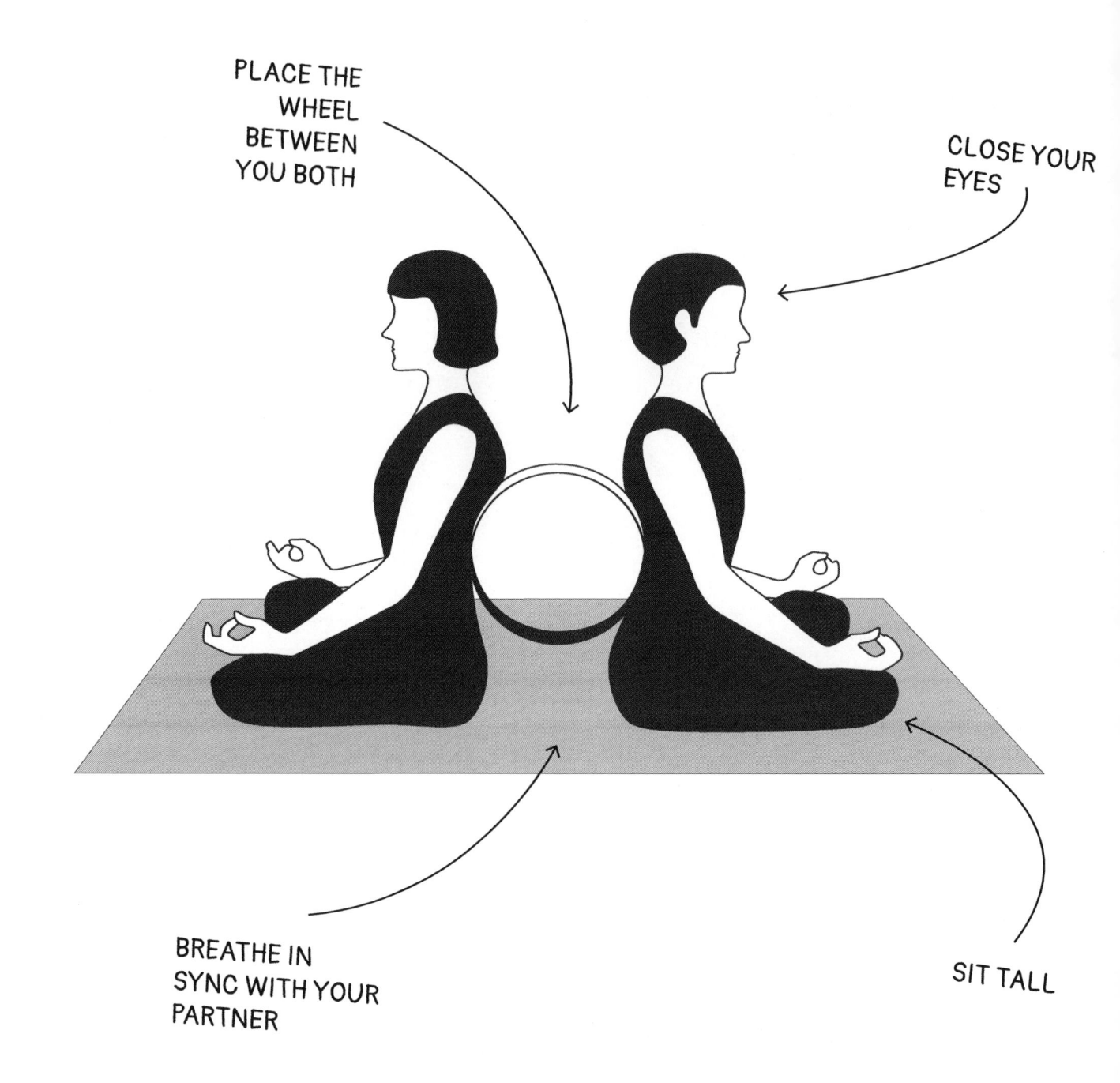

YOGA WHEEL BOOK

PLACE THE WHEEL BETWEEN YOU BOTH

CLOSE YOUR EYES

BREATHE IN SYNC WITH YOUR PARTNER

SIT TALL

Seated Meditation

Sukhasana

Practising Seated Meditation with a partner can help you to focus on your posture and breathing. By also including the wheel in this pose you both have a prompt to keep still, so that it doesn't fall.

1. Start in a seated position with your legs crossed and your back to your partner.

2. Place the wheel in between you both, so that it rests in the middle of your back.

3. Close your eyes and relax as you try to breathe in sync with your partner.

TARGETS: POSTURE, FOCUS

Follow us on Instagram

@yogawheel

Use our hashtag to get featured #yogawheel

We would love to see you using this book!
Tag @yogawheel in your photos

Printed in Great Britain
by Amazon